I0705413

ISBN: 9798670266925

TOTAL FITNESS

U.K. Edition

For Women

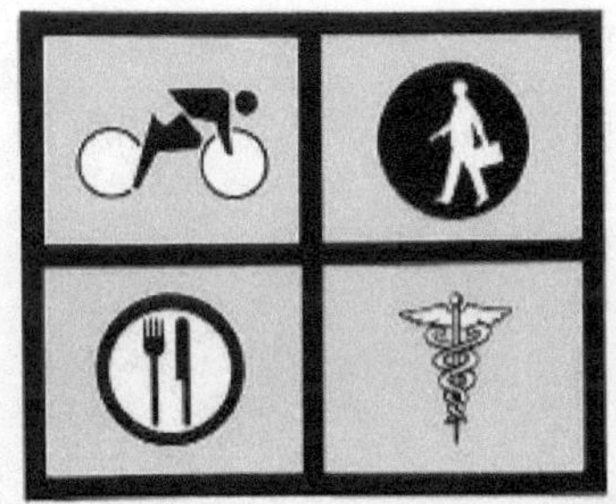

Vincent W. Antonetti, Ph.D.

NoPaperPress™

CONTENTS

LIST OF TABLES

LIST OF FIGURES

1. BEING FIT IS IMPORTANT

The person we call moderately active today, that is someone who walks an hour everyday and engages in some sport on the weekend, would have been considered sedentary a century ago! In many countries, the general lack of fitness of countless adults, who begin to show signs of old age – shortness of breath, obesity and clogged arteries – years earlier than their counterparts of just a few generations ago, is considered a national problem. The unfit person, who wants to call it a day two hours before quitting time and is obsessed with minor aches and pains, often lacks the vigour and physical toughness to cope with the long hours and high-stress that are part of the 21st century. The fit person, on the other hand, typically has greater energy, tackles problems and projects head on, gets more done in less time, is better able to cope with stress, has a positive approach that is contagious, and does not get sick as often.

In our view, for a person to fully enjoy life he or she must manage their health as effectively as they manage the other aspects of their life - and that this is best done using tried and true management techniques: first, define the problem; second, obtain the relevant facts; third, formulate an action plan; and last, make it happen! That is precisely the approach taken in this book. The intent here is to provide in a relatively complete form the facts needed for an in-depth understanding of all the components of a physical fitness program, and then to demonstrate how the information can be used to plan and implement a successful personal fitness program. All areas of fitness are covered: exercise, nutrition and weight control. To do this in the most efficient manner, the following pages are organized along the lines of a fitness handbook - with the emphasis on facts not frills - and all with the busy adult in mind.

Medical personnel, health education specialists, personal fitness trainers, and corporate fitness directors should find the data in this edition even more useful in devising or supervising physical fitness programmes. Whether this book is used as a professional reference, or as a personal fitness guide, the aim is to provide the facts and data needed to achieve and maintain a healthful physical fitness level.

Four of the leading causes of death in many industrialized countries are heart disease, cancer, stroke and diabetes. That's the bad news. The good news is that research indicates that people who exercise regularly, who eat the right foods and who maintain a normal weight, i.e., who are physically fit, can reduce their risk of heart attack, stroke and diabetes, and also gain some protection against certain forms of cancer.

Cardiovascular System

International cardiovascular disease statistics show that heart attacks prematurely claim the lives of more than 7-million people worldwide every year, surprisingly almost half are women, and many of the victims are relatively young. Because of this, some knowledge of the workings and diseases of the cardiovascular system is appropriate before we begin to discuss physical fitness.

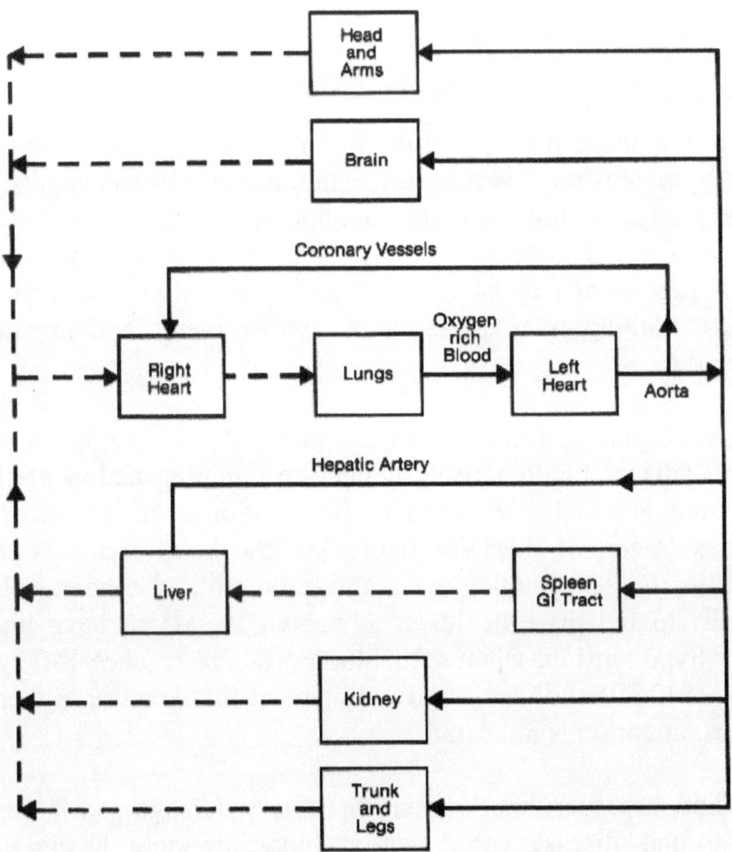

Figure 1.1: Block Diagram of Cardiovascular System

As illustrated in Figure 1.1, the cardiovascular system consists of the blood vessels through which blood flows and the heart which produces this flow. Beating about 72 times per minute, the average heart pumps approximately 60 millilitres of blood per beat, which results in a blood flow rate of about four litres per minute. The left side of the heart discharges oxygen-rich blood through the arteries bringing nourishment and oxygen to the body's cells. After waste gases such as carbon dioxide are removed from the cells, veins return the blood to the right side of the heart. The heart then pumps the blood to the lungs where carbon dioxide is removed and oxygen is absorbed from the air we breathe. The cycle is completed as the left side of the heart receives this oxygen-rich blood. When something goes wrong with the system, the condition is called cardiovascular disease.

Cardiovascular disease comes in many forms: the heart muscle itself can fail or become infected; valves can leak or refuse to close when they should; the timing mechanism can become erratic; but the most pervasive killers are high blood pressure and atherosclerosis.

High Blood Pressure

Recognized as a health problem of the first magnitude, high blood pressure – also called hypertension – is the most common cardiovascular disease. The World Health Organization estimates that 600 million people worldwide have high blood pressure. The dangers of high blood pressure include heart failure, heart attack, rupture of major blood vessels in the brain (stroke) and in other body organs, clotting in major arteries, eye problems and impairment of kidney function.

Simply stated, blood pressure is the force per unit area exerted by the blood against the walls of blood vessels under the pumping action of the heart. Blood pressure is usually recorded as two readings: an upper, or systolic figure, and a lower, or diastolic figure. As the heart contracts the blood pressure rises to the systolic level, and each time the heart relaxes the pressure falls to the diastolic level. A person is said to have high blood pressure, or hypertension, when their blood pressure reaches 140 systolic or 90 diastolic (140/90) and persistently remains at that level or higher. At this point medical attention is indicated.

Recent studies, however, have shown that artery damage and increased risk of cardiovascular disease can begin at blood pressure levels that were previously thought to be normal. The United States National Heart, Lung and Blood Institute now uses the term "prehypertension," defined as blood pressure that is 120 to 139 millimetres of mercury systolic or 80 to 90 millimetres of mercury systolic diastolic. This new category includes approximately 400 million more people world wide. The National Heart, Lung and Blood Institute's position is that people with blood pressure readings in this range do not have high blood pressure yet and do not need to take medication - but are likely to develop high blood pressure and should try to lower their pressure through lifestyle changes, such as a change in diet, exercise or losing weight.

Approximately 85 percent of those diagnosed with high blood pressure have what is called "primary hypertension," also called "essential hypertension." This designation refers to the group of hypertension cases for which there is no apparent explanation. If left untreated, primary hypertension greatly increases the risk that other cardiovascular diseases will occur. Although there is no cure for primary hypertension, it can be controlled – most often with medication.

The remaining 15 percent of those with high blood pressure have what is called "secondary hypertension." This form of high blood pressure can be attributed to a specific cause, such as clogged arteries or kidney disease. If the underlying cause of secondary hypertension can be diagnosed and eliminated, often secondary hypertension can be cured.

In most cases high blood pressure is painless and produces no symptoms. If symptoms do occur, they are similar to those caused by a myriad of other disorders. Because of this, even though high blood pressure is quite prevalent, it is discovered most often during the course of a periodic medical examination.

Some cases of hypertension can be managed effectively through a change in diet alone - without drugs. For the overweight, physicians first usually recommend a reducing diet. This is because the heart of an obese person is strained, being forced to pump more blood volume through a much larger cardiovascular system. Most medical doctors also urge that salt, more properly sodium, be restricted to curb the body's retention of fluid, thereby decreasing the volume of blood that must be pumped. If lifestyle changes fail to reduce a person's blood pressure, medication is usually prescribed.

Atherosclerosis

The narrowing and blocking of the blood vessels by the build-up of fatty deposits and other materials is called atherosclerosis, also known as hardening of the arteries.

The heart is a muscle and needs blood to survive. Narrowing of the blood vessels to the point where there is a decrease in the blood supply to the heart can cause angina (chest pain). The total absence of flow in a coronary artery leading to the heart, called a coronary occlusion or a coronary thrombosis, can damage or cause the death of a piece of the heart muscle, which cardiologists call a myocardial infarction or heart attack.

Heart Attack Warning Signs

- Prolonged, oppressive pain or unusual discomfort in the centre of your chest.

- Pain may spread to your shoulder, arm, neck or jaw, and sweating, nausea, vomiting and shortness of breath may ensue.

Sometimes the symptoms subside, then return. If you experience any of these warning signs, it is important to act quickly. If a medical doctor is not immediately available, get to a hospital emergency room at once.

Cardiovascular Disease Risk Factors

The rate of cardiovascular disease in the United States is much higher than that of most industrialized nations, with the death rate for men ages 45 to 54 years being the second highest among the world's most prosperous countries. As a result, approximately sixty years ago the United States government financed "Framingham Study" began tracking thousands of people and demonstrated a clear statistical association between cardiovascular disease and a number of "risk factors." These risk factors have been found time and time again in the history of thousands of people who have had heart attacks.

First, there are the risk factors we cannot control: gender and heredity. The data clearly show that men have heart attacks earlier and more frequently than women; that women are almost immune to heart attacks until past menopause; that individuals with a family history of premature heart disease have a far greater risk than those whose ancestors lived to a ripe old age; and that diabetes (left untreated) increases the danger of heart disease.

The **risk factors** often attributed to our lifestyle and, therefore, under our control - at least to some extent – are in approximate order of importance:

- **High blood pressure left untreated.**

- **Cigarette smoking.**

- **High blood cholesterol and other blood fats.**

- **Obesity.**

- **Lack of physical activity.**

- **A high-pressure existence.**

No one of these factors can be called the single cause of cardiovascular disease. Indeed studies show that a combination of risk factors dramatically increases the danger.

Stroke

Although some cells in the body can survive for as long as fifty minutes without blood, if the flow to the brain is cut off for ten or twenty seconds unconsciousness will occur, and deprived of blood circulation for four minutes or more results in brain damage. Blockage of the blood vessels leading to the brain or in the brain itself (sometimes a manifestation of atherosclerosis, other times caused by a clot) is called stroke.

Stroke Warning Signs

- Sudden numbness or weakness of the face, arm or leg, especially on one side

- Sudden headache, confusion, trouble speaking or understanding

- Sudden trouble seeing in one or both eyes

- Sudden trouble walking, dizziness, loss of balance or coordination

Stroke and cardiovascular disease have a lot in common: High blood pressure is an important cause of both illnesses, and many of the preceding cardiovascular disease risk factors also apply to stroke.

Diabetes

With the ranks of the obese increasing dramatically, the incidence of diabetes is reaching epidemic proportions in many industrialized countries. In 2002,

diabetes was the fifth leading cause of non-accidental death in the United States. Type 2 diabetes is the most common form. Previously called adult-onset diabetes, type-2 diabetes can begin at any age. It usually starts with insulin resistance, a condition in which fat, muscle, and liver cells do not use insulin properly. Being overweight and inactive (read unfit) increases your chance of developing type 2 diabetes.

What Can be Done?

It is not possible stop cardiovascular disease, heart attacks, stroke and diabetes completely, but enough is known to prevent many – if not most – premature incidents. In the pages that follow, a program will be outlined with a fitness prescription that is remarkably simple.

(Note, the cancer battle is not as straight forward. Substantial evidence indicates the fitness prescription that reduces the risk of cardiovascular disease, stroke and diabetes also exhibits a benefit against certain malignancies, such as colon cancer and breast cancer, and a promising benefit against others, but offers no protection with regard to many other cancers.)

➡ Note that the material in this book is not intended as a substitute for medical counselling. Everyone should have a medical check-up before beginning a physical fitness program (whether the program involves weight loss, nutritional changes, or exercise). And the physician conducting the medical exam should be made aware of and should approve the specific physical fitness routine planned. Further, the reader is cautioned that all fitness programmes include some risk of injury or illness.

2. FITNESS PRESCRIPTION

The physical conditions and living habits that increase the risk of premature heart disease and stroke have been identified, but for every risk there is a counteracting step you can take. Said another way, to reduce your risk you need to look at your entire way of living and in some instances rearrange your priorities.

No one set of rules will guarantee health or fitness. Age, gender, and physical condition are all factors in determining the specific programme that is best for you. We can delineate, however, the general guidelines for a total programme:

- **Have periodic medical checkups.**

- **Do not smoke.**

- **Practice good nutrition habits.**

- **Exercise regularly.**

- **Maintain a proper weight level.**

- **Learn to relax.**

- **Drink alcoholic beverages in moderation – if at all.**

Do Not Smoke

In many countries a pack of cigarettes carries a warning that cigarette smoking is dangerous to your health! These facts are not disputed: Nicotine and carbon monoxide in tobacco smoke are pathologically related to cardiovascular disease; and that tar collects in the pulmonary passages leading the way to emphysema and cancer. Clearly, tobacco and physical fitness are mutually exclusive. Undoubtedly one of the best things you can do for your body is to stop smoking.

Learn to Relax

Some researchers contend that the greatest single contributor to the development of coronary risk factors is the presence of a TYPE-A, "coronary personality." Such individuals are aggressive, competitive, compulsive, impatient, work additive and frequently anxious. These obsessions can lead to excessive social drinking - and often to domestic turmoil.

It is not easy to avoid stressful situations in the pressure-cooker world that is the 21st century. Although some stress is a normal, even a healthy part of living, sometimes you may get so keyed up by work or worry that you simply cannot relax. When this happens, you need a calming regulator for your emotions. Some people have a built in defence that says "Cool It!" Others may benefit from a change of pace, such as a workout at the gym, a brisk walk, or a relaxing talk with a friend or advisor.

The Benefits of Being Fit

Although our primary aim is to reduce the risk of cardiovascular illness, stroke, cancer and diabetes, physical fitness is much more than not being sick or merely being well. It is a positive quality. Ideally, it is the ability to withstand stress, and to persevere under circumstances where an unfit person would quit.

While the results will differ from individual to individual, most often **being fit will result in a longer life expectancy, less illness, a healthful appearance, the ability to work (and play) with vigour and an energy reserve for emergencies.**

After a prolonged period of sedentary living, people who undertake a physical fitness programme and attain a heightened level of fitness, report a dramatic reduction in chronic fatigue, an improved ability to relax, more energy for day-to-day tasks, firmer muscles and increased strength. In short, they feel better and look better too!

Everyone knows regular exercise improves your strength and flexibility and can help you lose weight. But did you know that regular exercise promotes the lose of fat rather than muscle and other non-fat tissue? Research also shows that people who include regular exercise as part of their weight-lose programme are more likely to keep off the weight they have lost than people who only changed their diet.

Not so evident, but perhaps even more important, are the beneficial changes in the functioning of the heart, lungs and circulatory system. Physical activity lowers your risk of developing heart disease and helps control blood pressure and diabetes. In addition, the old-fashioned idea that exercise is bad for the heart has been shown to be without scientific foundation. The heart is a pump

made of muscle. Just as exercise strengthens the other muscles in your body, it also strengthens your heart. With exercise your heart beat becomes stronger and steadier, breathing becomes deeper, and circulation improves.
In more specific terms, a well-designed total fitness programme - encompassing exercise, nutrition and weight control – will:

- Help you lose weight

- Lower your blood pressure

- Make your heart stronger and more efficient

- Keep your arteries supple and young

- Speed up your metabolism

- Convert fat to muscle

- Make your muscles larger with more definition - and more powerful

- Strengthen your bones

In addition, being fit will also reduce your risk of:

- Cardiovascular disease

- Stroke

- High blood pressure

- Diabetes

- Certain cancers

- Osteoporosis and bone fractures

Longevity: Being fit can't quite turn back the clock but it can make you look and feel younger than your chronological age – and you will probably live longer too. There are a number of scientific studies that have concluded that regular exercise reduces the hardship of illness and disability in old age and actually prolongs life by more than two years when compared to sedentary individuals. In fact, according to the Harvard School of Public Health, your life expectancy increases about two hours for every hour of regular exercise. So we should add the following to our list of benefits of being fit:

- You will look and feel younger than your chronological age.

- You will probably live longer – if you are physically fit.

Knowledge is a Requirement for Success

Certainly, the desire to be fit and the discipline to start and stay on a fitness programme are crucial. But along with desire and discipline, it is our belief that **only an in-depth understanding of weight control, nutrition and exercise will lead to long-term success**. As is true with many important and complex subjects, to achieve you need more than rules – you need solid understanding.

We leave motivation to others. Our mission is to impart the facts, data, knowledge and the systematic approach needed for enduring physical fitness. So take the time to read what follows. The reward will last you a lifetime.

3. FITNESS ASSESSMENT

Stated or not, everyone has goals in mind when they embark on a physical fitness programme. It could be reducing the risk of illness, losing weight, or becoming stronger. Before you begin your programme, however, you should know where you stand, i.e., your current fitness level. Assessing your current level in areas such as aerobic (cardio) capacity, strength, flexibility, body-fat, and even how appropriate your nutritional practices are, will help you establish what you should emphasize in your physical fitness programme and help you set goals.

Medical Assessment

In our opinion, everyone should have a medical assessment, or exam, before starting a physical fitness programme. The medical check-up may be as simple as a visit to a physician who is familiar with your medical history, or it may be a thorough physical exam.

Note, in all cases the physician conducting the medical exam should be made aware of and should approve the specific physical fitness programme you are planning. In addition, if you have or suspect you have cardiovascular disease or other health problems, if you are obese, if you have been totally inactive, or if you are 40 or older, before embarking on a physical fitness programme you should have a stress test supervised by a physician. Specific age-dependent guidelines are as follows:

Ages 20-29: For most young people in this age group a medical check-up will probably be a rather quick, basic medical exam.

Ages 30-39: The medical exam is somewhat more extensive for this age group and should include a resting EKG.

Ages 40-59: Those in this age category should proceed with still more care by having an exercising or stress-type EKG as part of their medical exam.

Ages 60 +: The medical check-up for people in this category is basically the same as for the 40-59 year olds.

To repeat, in all cases the physician conducting the medical exam should be made aware of and should approve the specific physical fitness routine you are planning. Some gyms, health clubs and fitness centres offer a complete fitness evaluation where your aerobic capacity, strength, flexibility and body-fat percentage are determined before you sign on to a programme. Besides being a good indicator of what sort of shape you are in, these tests give you a baseline you can use to judge your progress after some time on a fitness programme.

Alternatively, you can also get a good indication of your overall condition by taking some body measurements and performing a few simple tests as outlined in the following pages.

Aerobic-Capacity Assessment

A good measure of aerobic capacity, or cardio-respiratory fitness, is the volume of oxygen per minute per kilogram of body weight (called VO_{2max}) a person can process during hard exercise. Higher values of VO_{2max} indicate better aerobic fitness. For example, a 25 year-old man in excellent physical condition can process about 50 millilitres of oxygen per minute per kilogram of body weight; compared to less than 20 mL/min/kg for a 70 year-old woman in poor condition.

One of the best self assessment tests for VO_{2max} is the <u>Rockport Walking Test</u>. This is a field test, not a laboratory test, and consists of walking one mile (1609 metres) as rapidly as possible. At the end of the test you record your pulse and the time required to complete the walk. You then convert the time to completion and your pulse into VO_{2max} using the formulae (on the following page). Lastly, you enter Table 3.1 (also on the next page) with your calculated VO_{2max} and determine your cardio-respiratory fitness level.

There is some risk if you take the Rockport Fitness Walking Test without prior conditioning. That is why the following precautions are suggested.

1) Be sure to have a medical examination before taking the walking test.

2) If you are over 30 years old, postpone the walking test until you have been exercising regularly for at least one month.

3) You must be able to comfortably walk at least three kilometres before you take the walking test.

4) When you take the test, if you feel exhausted, experience shortness of breath, become dizzy or light headed, or nauseous, stop the test. Do not attempt a retest until you have exercised regularly for at least another three months, when your fitness level should have improved.

The One-Mile (1609 metre) Walking Test: If available, walk on a track or a measured and marked flat trail with a smooth surface. You also can use a treadmill. Although not as accurate, if need be you can walk on a street course you have driven and measured.

Before you start the test, warm up for several minutes with easy walking and stretching. Rest for about one minute. Then start the test. Walk as briskly as possible for 1609 metres, but remember you'll probably walk at least 12 minutes, so don't start too fast. Pick up the pace on the last 400 metres if you still feel strong. When you finish the test, it's important to immediately measure your pulse. (See page 50 for recommended pulse measurement techniques.)

At the conclusion of the test, you should feel slightly winded, but you should not be gasping for air. Your goal is to end the test feeling tired but not exhausted. Remember to cool down by continuing to walk slowly for a few minutes.

Gender	Age	Cardio-Respiratory Fitness Level			
		Poor	Fair	Good	Excellent
Men	20-29	33.0 - 36.4	36.5 - 42.4	42.5 - 46.4	46.5 - 52.4
	30-39	31.5 - 35.4	35.5 - 40.9	41.0 - 44.9	45.0 - 49.4
	40-49	30.2 - 33.5	33.6 - 38.9	39.0 - 43.7	43.8 - 48.0
	50-59	26.1 - 30.9	31.0 - 35.7	35.8 - 40.9	41.0 - 45.3
	60+	20.5 - 26.0	26.1 - 32.2	32.3 - 36.4	36.5 - 44.2
Women	20-29	23.6 - 28.9	29.0 - 32.9	33.0 - 36.9	37.0 - 41.0
	30-39	22.8 - 26.9	27.0 - 31.4	31.5 - 35.6	35.7 - 40.0
	40-49	21.0 - 24.4	24.5 - 28.9	29.0 - 32.8	32.9 - 36.9
	50-59	20.2 - 22.7	22.8 - 26.9	27.0 - 31.4	31.5 - 35.7
	60+	17.5 - 20.1	20.2 - 24.4	24.5 - 30.2	30.3 - 31.4

Table 3.1: VO_{2max} versus Fitness Level

Calculating VO_{2max}:   The following is undoubtedly the most difficult computation in this book, because VO_{2max} is a function of so many variables: gender, weight, age, heart rate and time to complete the test walk. Although the formulae are relatively complex, we have tried to simplify the calculation as much as possible.

The formula for women is: $VO_{2max} = 133 - W - H - A - T$

The formula for men is: $VO_{2max} = 139 - W - H - A - T$

where $W = 0.17 \times$ Weight (kg) $A = 0.39 \times$ Age
        $H = 0.157 \times$ Heart rate $T = 3.26 \times$ Time to walk 1609 metres

<u>Example 3.1</u>:   Determine VO_{2max} and the fitness level of a 29 year-old woman who weighs 10st 5lb (65.9 kilos). She finished the one-mile walking test (1609 metres) in 15 minutes and 30 seconds (which is 15.5 minutes) with a heart rate of 145 beats per minute.

The first step is to determine values for W, H, A and T.

   $W = 0.17 \times$ Weight $= 0.17 \times 65.9$ kg $= 11.20$

   $H = 0.157 \times$ Heart rate $= 0.157 \times 145$ beats/min $= 22.77$

   $A = 0.39 \times$ Age $= 0.39 \times 29$ years $= 11.31$

   $T = 3.26 \times$ Time $= 3.26 \times 15.5$ minutes $= 50.53$

Then calculate VO_{2max} using the formula for women.

   $VO_{2max} = 133 - W - H - A - T$
   $= 133 - 11.20 - 22.77 - 11.31 - 50.53 = 37.2$

Finally, enter Table 3.1 (on page 23) for a 29 year-old woman with $VO_{2max} = 37.2$ and find her fitness level is bordering on excellent.

Strength Assessment

Rather than the one repetition with maximum load strength-assessment approach, we prefer the much safer anaerobic muscular strength measuring technique, where your strength is assessed by the number of repetitions you can perform with a sub-maximal load. Moreover, in the tests that follow you will use your own body weight to determine how strong you are. The standard tests are: the press-up test, the sit-up test, and the squat test. Because the sit-up test can aggravate existing back problems, we only recommend the press-up and squat tests. The objective in both tests is see how many press-up and squat repetitions you can perform without stopping.

Press-up Test: For the test, men should execute the standard military press-up; i.e., your back and trunk should be rigid and straight and your weight should be supported by your arms and toes. Women should employ the familiar half press-up, supporting their weight with their arms and knees. Use Table 3.2 on the next page to assess your performance.

Squat Test: Stand with your back about 30 cm in front of a chair. Place your feet about shoulder width apart and extend your arms parallel to the floor to your front. Bend your knees and slowly lower your body until your butt just touches the seat of the chair. (But do not sit on the chair.) Then slowly return to the standing position. Repeat as often as you can without stopping. Use Table 3.3 on the next page to assess your performance.

Gender	Age	Press-up Performance		
		Below Average	Average	Above Average
Men	20-29	15 - 24	25 - 34	35 - 44
	30-39	10 - 19	20 - 29	30 - 34
	40-49	5 - 14	15 - 24	25 - 29
	50-59	0 - 9	10 - 19	20 - 24
	60-69	0 - 4	5 - 9	10 - 15
	70+	0 - 2	3 - 5	6 - 8
Women	20-29	0 - 16	17 - 33	34 - 50
	30-39	0 - 11	12 - 24	25 - 37
	40-49	0 - 7	8 - 19	20 - 29
	50-59	0 - 5	6 - 14	15 - 23
	60+	0 - 2	3 - 5	6 - 8

Table 3.2: Strength Assessment: Press-up Performance

Gender	Age	Squat-Test Performance		
		Below Average	Average	Above Average
Men	20-29	24 - 26	27 - 29	30 - 32
	30-39	21 - 23	24 - 26	27 - 29
	40-49	18 - 20	21 - 23	24 - 26
	50-59	15 - 17	18 - 20	21 - 23
	60+	12 - 14	15 - 17	18 – 20
Women	20-29	17 - 19	21 - 23	24 - 26
	30-39	15 - 17	18 - 20	21 - 23
	40-49	12 - 14	15 - 17	18 - 20
	50-59	9 - 11	12 - 14	15 - 17
	60+	6 - 8	9 - 11	12 - 14

Table 3.3: Strength Assessment: Squat Test Performance

Flexibility Assessment

Sit & Reach Test: This is a standard test to determine hip and trunk flexibility and is often used as a measure of overall flexibility. Remember to warm up with a few gentle stretches before you start the test. To conduct the test, tape a metre stick to the floor at the 23-cm mark. Remove your shoes and sit on the floor, with your legs forward and fully extended, so that the metre stick is between and almost parallel to your extended legs. (The metre stick's zero mark should be closest to you). Locate your heels at the 23-cm mark and move your feet about 25 cm apart. Place one hand over the other and slowly stretch forward (without jerking or bouncing), and extend the tips of your fingers as far as possible along the metre stick. Repeat three times. Your score is the furthest or highest number you are able to reach. Use Table 3.4 to assess your flexibility.

Body-Weight Assessment

Most people want to know what their proper or "best" body weight should be. Your weight as measured on a bathroom scale, however, can actually be misleading and certainly does not tell the whole story. The typical human body is a combination of bones, ligaments, tendons, organs, fluids, muscle and fat. When you lose or gain weight both your overall weight as well as the ratio of these components to one another changes.

Gender	Age	Sit & Reach Test Performance		
		Below Average	Average	Above Average
Men	20-29	10.3 - 18.9	19.0 - 28.1	28.2- 37.0
	30-39	9.0 - 17.7	17.8 - 26.8	26.9 -35.7
	40-49	7.8 - 16.4	16.5 -25.5	25.6 -34.4
	50-59	6.5 - 15.1	15.2 - 24.3	24.4 - 33.2
	60+	0 – 10.0	10.1 - 20.5	20.6 – 30.6
Women	20-29	21.7 - 29.1	29.2 - 37.0	37.1 - 44.6
	30-39	19.2 - 26.6	26.7 - 34.4	34.5 - 42.1
	40-49	10.3 - 21.5	21.6 - 33.2	33.3 - 40.8
	50-59	10.3 - 21.5	21.6 – 29.4	29.5 - 37.0
	60+	10.3 - 20.2	20.3 - 28.1	28.2 - 35.7

Table 3.4: Flexibility Assessment: Sit & Reach Test

Exercise physiologists consider the quantity of body fat compared to total body weight a critical measure of fitness, and contend, from the standpoint of good health. Table 3.5 shows the age-adjusted fat percentage for men and women men should have no more

	Age	Underweight	Healthy	Overweight	Obese
Men	**20 - 40**	Less than 8 %	8 – 19 %	19 – 25 %	Over 25 %
	41 - 60	Less than 11 %	11 – 22 %	22 – 27 %	Over 27 %
	61 - 80	Less than 13 %	13 – 25 %	25 – 30 %	Over 30 %
Women	**20 - 40**	Less than 21 %	21 – 33 %	33 – 39 %	Over 39 %
	41 - 60	Less than 23 %	23 – 35 %	35 – 40 %	Over 40 %
	61 - 80	Less than 24 %	24 – 36 %	36 – 42 %	Over 42 %

Table 3.5: Age-Adjusted Body Fat Percentage for Men & Women*

* Source: Gallagher et al., Am J Clin Nut 2000; 72:694-701

Percent body fat is estimated in a number of ways. The most accurate, used in many research laboratories, involves underwater or hydrostatic weighing to determine body density from which the percentage of body fat can be computed. The body fat percentage (and fitness) of many professional athletes is measured by under-water weighing. Lately, obesity researchers have started to use bioelectrical impedance testing and magnetic resonance imaging to measure body fat. None of these methods, however, are practical for personal use, and more convenient means have been devised whereby body fat can be estimated. For more information and tables to determine body fat percentage see Professional Weight Control for Men and Professional Weight Control for Women published by NoPaperPress. Both books have age-related body fat percentages and maximum and optimum waist sizes for men and women.

More recently, physicians and some scientists use a parameter called the Body Mass Index, or BMI, to determine if a person is overweight. The BMI takes into account both a person's weight and height and is calculated by dividing a person's weight in kilograms by their height in meters squared. Scientists categorize a man or woman's weight profile (Table 3.7) as a function of BMI. For readers living in the UK, Table 3.6 allows the determination of the BMI using body weight in stones and height in centimeters.

Weight (st.)	- Height (cm.) -									
	155	160	165	170	175	180	185	190	195	200
7	18.5									
8	21.2	19.9	18.7							
9	23.8	22.4	21.0	19.8	18.7					
10	26.5	24.8	23.4	22.0	20.8	19.6	18.6			
11	29.1	27.3	25.7	24.2	22.8	21.6	20.4	19.4	18.4	
12	31.8	29.8	28.0	26.4	24.9	23.6	22.3	21.1	20.1	19.1
13	34.4	32.3	30.4	28.6	27.0	25.5	24.2	22.9	21.7	20.7
14	37.1	34.8	32.7	30.8	29.1	27.5	26.0	24.7	23.4	22.3
15	39.7	37.3	35.0	33.0	31.2	29.4	27.9	26.4	25.1	23.9
16	42.4	39.8	37.4	35.2	33.2	31.4	29.7	28.2	26.8	25.4
17	45.0	42.2	39.7	37.4	35.3	33.4	31.6	30.0	28.4	27.0
18	47.7	44.7	42.0	39.6	37.4	35.3	33.4	31.7	30.1	28.6
20				44.0	39.5	39.3	39.0	35.2	33.5	31.8
22						43.2	40.9	38.8	36.8	35.0

Table 3.6: Body Mass Index (BMI) vs Height & Weight

BMI	Weight Profile
18.5 or less	Underweight
18.6 to 24.9	Normal
25.0 to 29.9	Overweight
30.0 to 39.9	Obese
40 or more	Extremely Obese

Table 3.7: Body Weight Profile

A more convenient way to use BMI is the New BMI-Based Weight vs. Height shown in Table 3.8, where the underweight category corresponds to BMI = 18.5 or less, normal BMI = 18.6 to 24.9, overweight BMI = 25.0 to 29.9, obese is BMI = 30.0 to 39.9 and extremely obese is BMI = 40 or more.

Height (cm)	Under (kg)	Normal (kg)	Over (kg)	Obese (kg)	Very Obese
150	41 or less	42 – 56	57 – 67	68 – 90	> 91
153	43 or less	44 – 58	59 – 70	71 – 93	> 94
156	45 or less	46 – 61	62 – 73	74 – 97	> 98
159	47 or less	48 – 63	64 – 76	77 – 101	> 102
162	49 or less	50 – 65	66 – 79	80 – 105	> 106
165	50 or less	51 – 68	69 – 81	82 – 109	> 110
168	52 or less	53 – 70	71 – 84	85 – 113	> 114
171	54 or less	55 – 73	74 – 87	88 – 117	> 118
174	56 or less	57 – 75	76 – 90	91 – 121	> 122
177	58 or less	59 – 78	79 – 94	95 – 125	> 126
180	60 or less	61 – 81	82 – 97	98 – 129	> 130
183	62 or less	63 – 83	84 – 100	101 – 134	> 135
186	64 or less	65 – 86	87 – 103	104 – 138	> 139
189	**140 or less**	67 – 89	90 – 107	108 – 143	> 144

Table 3.8: BMI-Based Weight vs. Height

Body-Weight Assessment Example

Example 3.2: Consider a woman who is 155 cm tall who weighs 90-kg (14 st 2 lbs). She has a 130 cm waist and her hip measures 111 cm. Determine her "best weight range" using two methods: a) BMI, Tables 3.6 and 3.7, b) Table 3.8, "BMI-Based Weight Range vs. Height."

a) <u>BMI Method</u>: Table 3.6 (on page 28) shows that at 155 cm and 90 kg her BMI = 37.5 and that she is without question obese. Table 3.7 also indicates that to get to the normal range, which requires a BMI of at most 24.9, but the standard BMI table (Table 3.6) does not indicate what she should weigh to be in the "normal" weight range.

b) <u>BMI-Based Weight Range vs. Height Table</u>: From Table 3.8 (on page 29), we note that for a 155 cm woman at 90 kg she is obese and would have to weigh between 45 and 60 kg to be deemed "normal weight."

Waist-to-Hip Ratio: Another very important weight-profile parameter is your waist-to-hip ratio. Health risks for heart attack and stroke increase considerably for men that have a waist to hip ratio greater than 1.0, and for women that have a waist to hip ratio greater than 0.8.

To calculate your ratio, measure your waist size (at its narrowest circumference) and divide it by your hip size (at the widest section). For example, a woman with a 130-cm waist and 111-cm hips would have a waist to hip ratio of 130/111 = 1.2, and would have an increased risk for a heart attack or stroke.

Nutrition Practices Assessment

Nutrition is normally not considered as part of a fitness assessment, but it is included here because it is a crucial and often overlooked element of a comprehensive physical fitness programme. To broadly assess how appropriate your current nutritional practices are please complete the following questionnaire. (You will need pencil and paper to keep your score.)

A. How many servings of vegetables do you eat in a typical day?

    1. None
    2. 1 serving
    3. 2 to 4
    4. 5 or more

B. How many servings of fruit do you usually eat in a day?

    1. None
    2. 1 serving
    3. 2 to 4
    4. 5 or more

C. How many servings of cereals and whole-grain bread do you eat in a typical day?

   1. None
   2. 1 serving
   3. 2 to 4
   4. 5 or more

D. How many times per week do you eat a fish or poultry?

   1. Never
   2. 1 time
   3. 2 to 3
   4. 4 times or more

E. How do you prepare and eat poultry?

   1. Fry & eat dark meat with skin & gravy
   2. Bake or broil & eat dark meat with skin & gravy
   3. Bake or broil & eat dark meat with skin removed
   4. Bake or broil & eat only white meat with skin removed

F. How many times per week do you eat beans, lentils, or peas?

   1. Never
   2. 1 time
   3. 2 to 3
   4. 4 times or more

G. How often do you eat meats like hamburger, salami, frankfurter, bacon, sausage?

   1. 7 or more times
   2. 4 to 6 times per week
   3. 2 to 3
   4. Rarely

H. When you consume milk, yogurt, ice cream, etcetera, you most often select:

   1. Only whole-fat dairy products
   2. Whole milk, but low-fat yogurt and ice cream
   3. Low-fat (1 or 2% fat)
   4. Skim or non-fat dairy products

I. If you were ordering potatoes in a restaurant would you choose:

1. Fried potatoes
2. Baked or boiled with butter and/or sour cream
3. Boiled without butter or sour cream
4. Baked without butter or sour cream

J. How many times per week do you eat at a fast-food restaurant?

1. 5 times or more
2. 3 or 4 times per week
3. 1 or 2
4. Rarely

K. How frequently do you add salt to your food after it is served?

1. At every meal
2. Once per day
3. 2 or 3 times per week
4. Rarely

L. How often do you eat sweets (candy bar, cookies, pastries, ice cream)?

1. More than one sweet per day
2. About one per day
3. 2 or 4 sweets per week
4. Rarely

M. Do you take any vitamin or mineral supplements?

1. None
2. Take "natural" herbal supplements
3. Take individual vitamins supplements (like C, E, etcetera)
4. Take multi-vitamin and mineral supplement

N. If you wanted to lose weight, how would you proceed?

1. Go on a "crash diet"
2. Stop eating carbohydrates
3. Cut back on carbohydrates & increase exercise
4. Reduce caloric intake (portion sizes) & increase exercise

This completes our brief nutrition practices assessment. Add up your score and see how you compare to the following standards.

Excellent = 49 to 56 points
Good = 41 to 48

Fair = 32 to 40
Poor = 23 to 31
Very Poor = 14 to 22

Time to Set Goals

To this point, in Chapter 1 we defined the problem; in Chapter 2 we outlined a "fitness prescription," and in Chapter 3 we briefly set forth techniques you can use to assess your aerobic capacity, your strength, your flexibility, your body weight, and your nutritional practices, i.e., your current total fitness level.

Now it's time to review your fitness-self-assessment test results and set some broad personal fitness goals, such as losing weight and improving your aerobic capacity. You're not quite ready to construct a total programme. That will have to wait until you read the exercise, nutrition and weight control chapters. These topics are somewhat complex and are treated in depth in the pages that follow.

4. EXERCISE BASICS

Many of us exist largely through mental efforts - by our wits and skill. All the advances of modern technology – from washing machines to automobiles to computers – have made life easier and physically much less demanding. For many people, the common tasks of living and working no longer provide enough exercise to develop and maintain cardiovascular and respiratory fitness and good muscle tone. With any luck we can go for weeks without working up a good sweat or drawing a deep breath! Our bodies, however, are virtually identical to that of primitive humans who survived through physical efforts – by strength and stamina.

In fact, the bodies we inherited are just not built to be immobile and passive. The sad fact, however, is that after years of education and information programmes by government agencies, medical associations and insurance companies relatively few people engage in regular planned exercise – despite the reality that we need to be active to keep our systems working efficiently and to rid ourselves of emotional tension.

There are two ways to become more physically active: 1) Increase the physical activity in your daily life; and 2) Start on a regular exercise programme. Better still would be a combination of both.

Be More Active Every Day

Before we address exercise programmes, here are some ways you can increase physical activity in your daily routine:

- Change your attitude toward the occasional "bothersome" physical tasks that you encounter in daily living. Consider anytime you have to lift, bend, reach, walk as an opportunity to burn additional calories and as an extension of your formal workout.

- Look for opportunities to walk, such as walking up stairs (two at a time if you can) rather than using an elevator, walking to a local store rather than driving, walking the course if you play golf, and mowing your lawn. At work stand up and stretch two or three times a day, read standing up, etcetera.

- Engage in leisure activities such as dancing, bowling and gardening more often. They can be enjoyable and provide added exercise.

Each of these daily activities taken alone may not seem like much, but done every day for many years they can add up to a considerable number of extra kcalories burned.

Energy Used During Different Activities

Table 4.1 (on the next page) shows the number of kcalories burned per hour for various activities. Although the data in the table are from reliable sources, you may detect that some of the values are at slight variance with those in other books. There are several reasons for this. First, the intensity of the activity being measured may actually vary (for example handball can be played at many different levels – with a different number of kcalories burned at each level). Then the energy expended by same weight subjects engaged in the same activity does vary somewhat; and finally measurement techniques and data collection accuracy vary slightly from laboratory to laboratory. The best one can do, therefore, is arrive at an average from the available data, which often requires judgment and compromise. More important, notice that the calories expended for a given activity depends on your weight. Good news: **For any activity, the more you weigh the more calories you burn!**

Energy Expended Example

Example 4.1:   Determine the number of kcalories burned by a 13st 7lb woman or man who walks 11 kilometres in two hours.

First calculate the person's walking speed = 11 km / 2 hours = 5.5 km/hr. Because 13st 7lb is not listed in Table 4.1 (on the next page), we use the neighboring value of 14 st. Then from Table 4.1 find that walking at 5.5 km/hr, a person weighing 14 stone burns 388 kcalories per hour. In two hours, therefore, a person weighing 14 stone would burn, 2 x 388 = 776 kcalories.

But from this we must subtract the number of calories a 14 stone person would have used anyway if, instead of walking, he or she just sat for the two hours. From Table 4.1 this amounts to 114 kcalories per hour, or 228 kcalories in two hours. Then the net energy a 14 stone person would expend walking (over and above just sitting) totals 776 − 228 = 548 kcalories. However, the individual in this example weighs 13st 7lb (13.5 stone) and would expend proportionately fewer calories than a person that weighs 14 stone, and therefore would burn: 548 x 13.5 / 14 = <u>528 kcalories</u>

Activity	Weight (Stone)								
	9	10	11	12	13	14	16	18	20
Aerobics (dance)	516	573	630	687	745	802	917	1031	1146
Basketball	401	445	490	534	579	623	712	801	890
Bicycling (13 mph)	458	508	559	610	661	712	814	915	1017
Cycling (stationary)	401	445	490	534	579	623	712	801	890
Cricket	284	315	347	378	410	441	504	567	630
Dancing (ballroom)	262	292	321	350	379	408	466	525	583
Golf (pulling cart)	284	315	347	378	410	441	504	567	630
Golf (riding cart)	199	222	244	266	288	310	354	399	443
Handball	384	426	469	512	554	597	682	768	853
Hiking	336	373	411	448	486	523	598	672	747
Hockey (ice/field)	451	502	552	602	652	702	802	903	1003
Horseback riding	226	251	276	301	326	351	401	451	501
Jogging	714	793	873	952	1032	1111	1270	1428	1587
Mowing lawn	314	349	384	419	454	489	559	629	699
Raking leaves	345	383	421	459	498	536	613	689	766
Rowing (moderate)	399	443	488	532	577	621	710	798	887
Sitting	73	82	90	98	106	114	130	147	163
Skating	399	443	488	532	577	621	710	798	887
Skiing (+ country)	457	508	559	609	660	711	813	914	1016
Skiing (downhill)	347	385	424	462	501	539	616	693	770
Skipping rope	480	533	587	640	694	747	854	960	1067
Soccer (football)	431	479	526	574	622	670	766	861	957
Softball	284	315	347	378	410	441	504	567	630
Squash	384	426	469	512	554	597	682	768	853
Swimming laps	462	513	565	616	668	719	822	924	1027
Tennis (singles)	336	373	411	448	486	523	598	672	747
Tennis (doubles)	255	283	311	339	368	396	453	509	566
Walking (4.8 kph)	204	227	249	272	294	317	362	408	453
Walking (5.5 kph)	249	277	305	333	360	388	443	499	554
Walking (6.5 kph)	317	353	387	423	458	493	563	634	704

Table 4.1: Energy Expended (kcal per hour) for Different Activities

Types of Exercise

Simply stated there are **three basic types of exercise: aerobic, stretching, and strengthening**.

1) **Aerobic exercises** (also called "cardio") condition your cardiovascular system. Aerobic exercises, such as jogging, swimming, cycling, brisk walking, skipping rope, jogging in place, and many others, are deep breathing and continuous, with rhythmic and repetitive contractions of your large muscle groups. Most aerobic exercises have one thing in common: they make you work hard and require that you process a great deal of oxygen.

   In fact, aerobic is a word derived from the Greek, meaning "with oxygen." Aerobic activities require oxygen for the production of energy. The main goal of an aerobic exercise programme is to increase the rate which your body can process oxygen, i.e., increase VO_{2max}. A well-conditioned person with efficient lungs and a strong heart can pump large volumes of blood, can breathe large volumes of air, and via the blood circulatory system effectively transport the oxygen in the air they breathe to all parts of their body.

   During aerobic exercise, the large muscles of the body continuously flood the heart with a great deal of blood; the heart beats faster; blood flow rate increases; and the lungs transport large quantities of oxygen to the blood. Regular exercise of this type "trains" the heart to pump more blood with less effort. Aerobic exercise improves the circulatory system by developing more elastic arteries and by creating peripheral or extra blood paths to the heart; and aerobic exercise strengthens the muscles of respiration increasing the volume of oxygen that can be processed within a given time. Done regularly, aerobic exercises improve stamina and endurance, and most importantly promote what should be your central exercise goal – cardiovascular fitness. For if your cardiovascular system is not in shape, you're not in shape – no matter how many press-ups or crunches you can do! In net, aerobic exercises develop a powerful heart, an effective circulatory system and efficient lungs.

   Aerobic exercises can be further subdivided according to how strenuous they are and how well they condition the heart and lungs. (Note, there are exercises other than those shown that could be included in the groupings that follow.)

Group A: Bicycling, Cross-country skiing, Dancing (aerobic), Hiking in rugged terrain, Ice Hockey, Jogging, Jogging in place, Rowing, Skipping rope, Stair climbing, and Stationary cycling.

Group B: Basketball, Field Hockey, Callisthenics, Handball, Racquetball, Skiing (downhill), Soccer (football), Squash, Tennis (singles), Volleyball, and Walking (briskly).

Group C: Badminton, Baseball, Bowling, Cricket, Dancing, Gardening, Golf (carrying or pulling clubs), Horseback riding, Housework, Ping-pong, Shuffleboard, Softball, and Walking (moderate to leisurely).

The vigorous exercises in Group A are intended for those already in good condition who want to further strengthen their heart and lungs and improve their aerobic capacity. The moderate exercises in Group B are not as demanding as those in Group A, but they are nevertheless good choices and can condition your heart and lungs. The exercises in Group C are actually not aerobic because they are either low intensity or not continuous, or both, but they still can be beneficial in that they improve muscle tone and coordination, relieve tension and burn some calories. (Note that some exercises in one group if done vigorously could easily be as demanding as those in the next higher grouping. For example, a very intense game of squash could move it from the Group B to the Group A category.)

As a final point, please note that the exercise portion of *Total Fitness* is aimed at the beginner who wants to improve her fitness level and general health, and also for someone who has already attained some degree of fitness but wants to learn more and go on to the next level. It is not intended for individuals who want to be highly-conditioned athletes and so topics such as interval, tempo and uphill training methods are not covered. (On the other hand, people at all fitness levels will find the information in Chapter 5 "Nutrition Basics" and especially in Chapter 6 "Weight Control" extremely valuable.)

2) **Stretching-type exercises** such as yoga, tai chi, Pilates and to a lesser extent callisthenics can improve your flexibility – and some of the exercises can make you somewhat stronger.

As you age you inevitably start to loose flexibility. Your gait becomes stiffer; you cannot stand quite as upright as you used to; it becomes tougher to bend over; and you have difficulty turning your neck. Regardless of your age, however, stretching can make you more flexible, less injury prone, and can reduce the pain and discomfort associated with tight muscles and shortened tendons. Realize, however, that stretching exercises do not condition your heart and lungs. Stretching exercises are fine as long as they are performed in addition to rather than in place of an aerobic exercise.

Most experts do recommend stretching before and after aerobic and strength routines. However, never stretch cold muscles and always do some form of warm up prior to stretching. Stretch slowly and hold gently. You should stretch to the point of feeling a gentle pull, but never to the point of feeling pain. And when you stretch – do not bounce.

3) **Muscle building and strengthening exercises,** e.g., weight lifting, use of exercise machines found in fitness centres and isometrics.

Once more, as you age you loose muscle mass, your bone density decreases and you lose strength. Exercises like weight lifting strengthen your muscles, bones and joints. Strengthening exercises also reduce your risk of developing osteoporosis, a severe bone-loss disease, which can lead to easily fractured bones and all the complications that often follow. Strong muscles not only allow you to lift a sleepy four-year old out of a car without difficulty and lug groceries up to second floor flat, but as with increased flexibility, strong muscles also make you less injury prone. **Strengthening exercises are beneficial and should be a part of your fitness routine, but again they should be performed in addition to an aerobic exercise** because alone they cannot condition your heart and lungs.

Select the Correct Activity

Selecting the right fitness activity is the key to a successful conditioning programme. You should try to pick an activity (or activities) you will enjoy. Factors to consider in choosing your activity are: your medical condition; your age; your fitness level; your exercise goals; your daily and overall schedule; exercise outdoors or indoors; exercise alone or with others; and how much money you are prepared to spend. You may decide to concentrate on one activity such as squash, or you may choose to walk briskly some days and lift weights on other days. Incidentally, three to five days of a vigorous aerobic exercise plus two days of either strength or flexibility exercises per week is a good combination. Whatever you settle on make sure it is an activity (or activities) that can be done regularly and that you enjoy.

Your Medical Condition: If you have a medical condition such as a heart problem, diabetes, osteoporosis, etcetera, or if you are a female who is pregnant or breast-feeding, you should proceed with caution, and be sure to talk to your doctor before you start any exercise activity.

Your Age: The age-dependent guidelines for how to proceed are as follows:

<u>Ages 20-29</u>: Assuming a clean bill of health from a medical exam, young men and women - unless badly overweight – can usually start an exercise programme immediately.

<u>Ages 30-39</u>: The precautions here are the same as for the 20-29 year-old age group except that the medical check-up should also include a resting EKG.

<u>Ages 40-59</u>: Those in this age category should proceed with still more care by having an exercising or stress-type EKG as part of their medical exam.

<u>Ages 60-up</u>: The medical check-up is the same as for the 40-59 year old group. (Unless one has been physically active for a number of years, most physicians feel that at this age exercise should be limited to walking and moderate flexibility and/or strengthening exercises to improve muscle tone.)

Your Fitness Level: If you have been inactive for some time, rather than starting with one of the more strenuous exercises, **beginners of all ages should initially confine themselves to walking** until they can easily walk about 3½ km at a brisk pace. When you reach this stage more strenuous exercises can be attempted if desired. Furthermore, some sports medicine physicians contend that **if you are badly overweight you should limit your exercise to walking** until you have lost weight to the point where you are less than 25 percent overweight. For example, a female who is 162 cm tall and weighs 14 stone, from Table 3.8 (on page 29), has to get to 65 kg (10 st 3 lbs or 143 lbs) to be considered "normal" weight. Twenty-five percent of 143 lbs is 36 lbs. Therefore, she should limit her exercise to walking until she has reduced her weight to less than (143 + 36), or about 12st 11lb.

Your Exercise Goals: If you want to strengthen your heart and lungs, improve your aerobic capacity and burn a lot of calories select an aerobic activity from Group A or B. If you want to improve your flexibility select a stretching type exercise. And if you want to become physically stronger choose one of the strength-building exercises.

Your Schedule: Only you know what the demands on your time from work, family and your social life are. What is the best time of day for you? Which days of the week best fit your schedule? Of course, you must be open to rearranging your priorities to fit exercise into your daily life.

Outdoors or Indoors: If you decide to exercise outdoors you should also have an alternate indoor activity, an activity you can fall back on in bad weather. For example, if you choose to jog outside early in the morning before work, you may want to purchase a treadmill for use at home on days when it is either too hot, too cold or the weather is bad.

Alone or with Others: On the plus side, an exercise partner can make exercise more enjoyable and can help you get going and keep going on days when you might otherwise quit. On the other hand, a partner probably means that you have the schedules of two busy people to contend with and plan around, which can at times actually hinder your workout.

How Much Money Are You Prepared to Spend: For many activities, you will need little or no special equipment. For instance, walking outside only requires comfortable shoes; whereas, joining and working out at a fitness centre can be relatively expensive.

Aerobic Exercise: How Hard?

Because cardiovascular fitness should be your prime concern, **the central part of your exercise programme should be an aerobic exercise done regularly**. Additional stretching and strengthening exercises should be included as time allows – but never to the exclusion of the aerobic portion of your programme.

An aerobic exercise routine should be vigorous enough to condition the cardiovascular system but not so strenuous as to exceed safe limits. Some experts define safe as an exercise pace that is "comfortable." What they mean is that if, for example, you are jogging or walking briskly you should be able to converse comfortably with a partner. They add that you should be breathing and feeling normally within ten minutes after you stop exercising. If not you are exercising too vigorously. Other signs that you are pushing too hard include difficulty breathing, feeling faint, or feeling weak - during or after exercising. If you experience any of these symptoms, you are exercising too intensely and you should cut back.

Others prefer a more quantitative definition. They refer to the beneficial yet safe exercise region as the "Target Training Zone," or TTZ, which is determined by monitoring your pulse. The idea is to raise your pulse through exercise to a specific range (the target training zone) and hold it there for an extended period to obtain a cardiovascular benefit. On this concept rests the so-called heart-rated theory of exercise, which relies on your heart rate (or pulse) to establish the proper exercise intensity.

Aerobic Exercise: Target-Training Zone

The **Target-Training Zone (TTZ) is a measure of aerobic exercise intensity**. Use the following procedure to calculate your individual target-training zone:

1) Calculate your **Maximum heart rate** = 220 – Age in years. (Your maximum heart rate is the fastest your heart can beat. You definitely must exercise well below this level.)

2) Compute your **Maximum heart rate reserve** = Maximum heart rate – Resting pulse.

3) Lastly, calculate your **TTZ** = (Maximum heart rate reserve multiplied by Exercise intensity level) + Resting pulse.

If you would rather not do the mathematics, you may determine your TTZ from Tables 4.2 and 4.3 (on pages 43 and 44). But before that, you need to determine the exercise intensity level that is right for you.

Aerobic Exercise: Intensity-Level Guidelines

Many exercise physiologists recommend the following guidelines:

- <u>Low Exercise-Intensity Level:</u> This intensity level should be used by anyone over 50 years old, and by those starting a physical fitness programme after many years of inactivity regardless of their age. People in this classification should begin exercising at 40 to 50% of their target-training zone (TTZ).

- <u>Moderate Exercise-Intensity Level:</u> This applies to moderately active people who are under 50 years old and who, for example, have been walking about 4 kilometres per day regularly. These men and women may begin exercising at 50 to 65% of their TTZ.

- <u>High Exercise Intensity Level:</u> This level applies to very active, well-trained, fit people under 50 years old. These individuals may exercise at 65 to 80% of their TTZ.

Keep in mind that these recommendations are aimed at the general population. In other words, they may not be right for you. Some people cannot raise their pulse, despite vigorous exercise, into their target-training zone. If you are one of these individuals, you probably have a maximum heart rate that is lower than average and so should disregard the target training zones shown here. Rather you should try to establish and be guided by a lower, more <u>comfortable</u>, more personal, exercising pulse range.

In addition, be aware that some blood pressure medications (such as beta-blockers) may lower your maximum heart rate and resting pulse. If you are taking blood pressure medication, consult your cardiologist for guidance before using the target training zone approach.

Age	Resting Pulse	Exercise Intensity (%)				
		40	50	60	70	80
20	50	110	125	140	155	170
	60	116	130	144	158	172
	70	122	135	148	161	174
	80	128	140	140	164	176
25	50	108	123	137	152	166
	60	114	128	141	155	168
	70	120	133	145	158	170
	80	126	138	149	161	172
30	50	106	120	134	148	162
	60	112	125	138	151	164
	70	118	130	142	154	166
	80	124	135	146	157	168
35	50	104	118	131	145	158
	60	110	123	135	148	160
	70	116	128	139	151	162
	80	122	133	143	154	164
40	50	102	115	128	141	154
	60	108	120	132	144	156
	70	114	125	136	147	158
	80	120	130	140	150	160

Table 4.2: Target-Training Zone: Ages 20 to 40 years

Age	Resting Pulse	Exercise Intensity (%)				
		40	50	60	70	80
45	50	100	113	125	138	150
	60	106	118	129	141	152
	70	112	123	133	144	154
	80	118	128	137	147	156
50	50	98	110	122	134	146
	60	104	115	126	137	148
	70	110	120	130	140	150
	80	116	125	134	143	152
55	50	96	108	119	131	142
	60	102	113	123	134	144
	70	108	118	127	137	146
	80	114	123	131	140	148
60	50	94	105	116	127	138
	60	100	110	120	130	140
	70	106	115	124	133	142
	80	112	120	128	136	144
65	50	92	103	113	124	134
	60	98	108	117	127	136
	70	104	113	121	130	138
	80	110	118	125	133	140

Table 4.3: Target-Training Zone: Ages 45 to 65 years

If you do use the target-training zone approach, your pulse becomes your exercise guide. In addition, after a couple of months of aerobic exercise a sure indication that you are rounding into shape, making progress, is that your resting pulse slows down somewhat – especially if it was relatively fast at the start. This is because well-conditioned strengthened hearts are more efficient and so beat more slowly at rest. Trained athletes often have a resting pulse of 50 beats per minute or lower, whereas the "average" pulse is 72 to 76 for untrained men and 75 to 80 for untrained women. Furthermore, as you become more physically fit you will have to exercise more vigorously to get your exercising pulse rate into your target-training zone.

Target-Training Zone Example

<u>Example 4.2</u>:   Determine the target-training zone (TTZ) for a 40-year old relatively inactive woman with a resting pulse of 70, whose physician has approved her intention to start an aerobic exercise programme.

Because she is relatively inactive but also relatively young, following the exercise-intensity level guidelines outlined earlier, she determines that she may start exercising at about 50 percent of her maximum heart rate reserve. She determines her (TTZ) as follows:

Maximum heart rate = 220 – Age in years = 220 – 40 = 180

Maximum heart rate reserve = Maximum heart rate – Resting pulse
= 180 – 70 = 110

TTZ = (Maximum heart rate reserve multiplied by Exercise intensity level) + Resting pulse

TTZ = (110 x 0.50) + 70 = <u>125 beats per minute</u>

(Note, the exercise-intensity level was converted from 50 % to the decimal equivalent 0.50.)

Alternatively, the 40-year old woman could have used Table 4.2, where first she would search the far left side of the table and locate her age (40). Then from the four possible resting pulse selections she would choose (70); finally she would run her finger horizontally (to the right) until she intersects the vertical column headed by the 50 percent exercise intensity level where she would find her TTZ of 125 beats per minute. Because it is difficult to get an exact pulse during or immediately after exercising and this is not an exact science, she should convert her calculated TTZ into a TTZ range. In this case, for a 50 percent exercise intensity level her TTZ range would be about 122 to 128 beats per minute.

When you cannot find your exact combination of age, resting pulse and exercise intensity level in tables 4.2 and 4.3, an estimating technique called interpolation[1] can be used to calculate your TTZ – although it would probably be easier for you to just use the formulae shown on page 42 and the mathematical procedure illustrated in Example 4.2.

---

2. A description of the mathematical procedure called interpolation is beyond the scope of this book.

Aerobic Exercise: How Long & How Often?

The American College of Sports Medicine recommends that an exercise heart rate of 60 to 90 percent of your maximum heart rate should be maintained for about 30 to 45 minutes three to five days per week to become reasonably fit. They also stated, "For most people exercising at the lower end of their heart rate range for a longer time is better than exercising at the higher end of the range for a shorter time." The United States Surgeon General recommends that people accumulate 30 minutes of moderate activity on most, if not all, days of the week. More recently, the Institute of Medicine suggested 60 minutes of moderate exercise every day. To confuse matters even more, many exercise physiologists favour the following exercise schedule:

- <u>Low Exercise-Intensity Level</u> (40 to 50% of maximum heart rate reserve):   People in this category (because of their age or lack of fitness) should work up to exercising 60 minutes per day at least five days per week. Despite the low intensity exercise level participants should achieve what exercise physiologists feel is an acceptable – albeit minimum – level of fitness.

- <u>Moderate Exercise-Intensity Level</u> (50 to 65% of maximum heart rate reserve): Men and women at this level should build up to 45 minutes of exercise per day at least five days per week to achieve a minimum fitness level.

- <u>High Exercise-Intensity Level</u> (65 to 80% of maximum heart rate reserve): In this category, individuals should work up to 30 minutes of exercise per day at least five days per week for a minimally acceptable fitness level.

As you can see, in general if you exercise at the lower exercise intensity levels your workout should last longer. Moreover, the longer and more frequently you exercise the greater your fitness reward. How fit you become is really a matter of your age, your genes, how fit you think you should be – and how hard you are willing to work. But do not overdo it! Again, it is worth repeating, everyone should have medical clearance before beginning any exercise programme.

Aerobic Exercise: Typical Workout

First, do not smoke before you exercise (or after for that matter); do not eat for two hours before you start exercising, and refrain from drinking any alcohol for four hours prior to beginning your exercise routine. A classic aerobic exercise routine consists of a warm up, your main exercise, and a cool down.

- Start with a three to seven minute warm up. Three minutes of stretching is sufficient if you are going to engage in a low intensity Group C exercise such as badminton; whereas a longer seven-minute warm up is better preparation for a high intensity Group A aerobic exercises such as jogging, cycling or stair climbing.

- Then move on to 30 to 60 minutes of your main aerobic exercise.

- Finish with a three to seven minute cool down period. Once more, if you are finishing a low-intensity exercise three minutes is enough. After a moderate or high-intensity aerobic exercise a seven minute cool down is more appropriate.

Warm up: Going from a resting state to a moderate or high-intensity exercise is a large disparity. The warm up period gives your body time to limber up, to bridge the gap and get ready for the more strenuous exercise to follow. Tension in your muscles and nerves is released; your large-frame muscles, ligaments and joints are stretched and put through their full range of motion; and your arteries and capillaries start to dilate as your heart beats faster and your blood flow rate increases.

Begin your warm up by walking slowly and gradually increase your pace as you approach the end of the warm up period. Next stretch. **Never stretch cold muscles**. Many stretches are based on yoga, where you start with good posture and then use your body weight to stretch your tissues. The following is a list of stretching exercises for your arms, neck, back and legs that are especially suited for warm up and cool down periods. Stretches (c) through (g) are illustrated in Figure 4.1, on page 49. (Some of these stretches can be done toward the end of the walking segment of your warm-up.) Perform the stretches as described.

a) <u>Neck Swivel</u>: From a standing position, with your arms hanging loosely, rotate your head about your neck, five times clockwise, then five times counter clockwise.

b) <u>Shoulder Roll</u>: While standing, with your arms hanging loosely at your side rotate your shoulders first in a forward motion, then backwards. Repeat five times.

c) <u>Arm Pumping</u>: Again, from a standing position, raise your elbows to shoulder height. Pull your elbows and arms slowly rearward as you thrust your chest forward. Repeat five times.

d) <u>Side to side Stretch</u>: From a standing position, raise both hands over your head. Bend slowly from side to side. Repeat five times.

e) <u>Toe Touch</u>: Sit along a bench and place your right leg on the bench. Position your left leg on the floor. Lean forward and try to touch your right toe until feel a stretch behind your right knee and calf. Do not bounce. Hold for a count of ten. Repeat with left leg raised. (This stretch can also be done from a standing position by placing a leg on a chair.)

f) <u>Wall Push to Stretch Calves</u>: Stand about two feet from a wall. Then as you extend your arms forward lean into the wall. Keep both heels flat on the floor. Do not bounce. Hold this position for a count of ten.

g) <u>Quad Stretch</u>: Balance yourself by placing your left hand on a wall. Bend your right leg and move your right heel toward your rear end. Grab your right foot with your right hand. Pull very gently. You should feel mild pressure in your right quad (the front of your right thigh). Do not bounce. Hold for a count of ten. Repeat for the left leg.

Do not feel limited to the following stretching exercises. There are many, many other good stretches available (too many to discuss here) that you might prefer.

If your main activity is a low-intensity exercise, you can conclude your warm up after stretching out. If you are going on to a moderate or high-intensity aerobic exercise, after stretching continue to your main aerobic exercise but at a relatively lower level. Over the next few minutes gradually increase the intensity so that your pulse approaches your target training zone. For instance, if you are a jogger you might warm up as follows: Start by walking slowly but steadily walk faster. After approximately five minutes stop and do two minutes of stretching. In theory, your warm up is over, but begin the main portion of your exercise by walking much faster, transition to a slow jog, then jog somewhat faster, and so on until, after about five minutes you have reached your regular jogging pace.

Main Exercise: Now you can begin your aerobic exercise of choice in earnest, stopping only to see that your pulse is in your target-training zone. If not, adjust your exercise level, exerting more or less effort. (Eventually, you will be able to sense that you are exercising at the correct intensity level and need only monitor your pulse occasionally.)

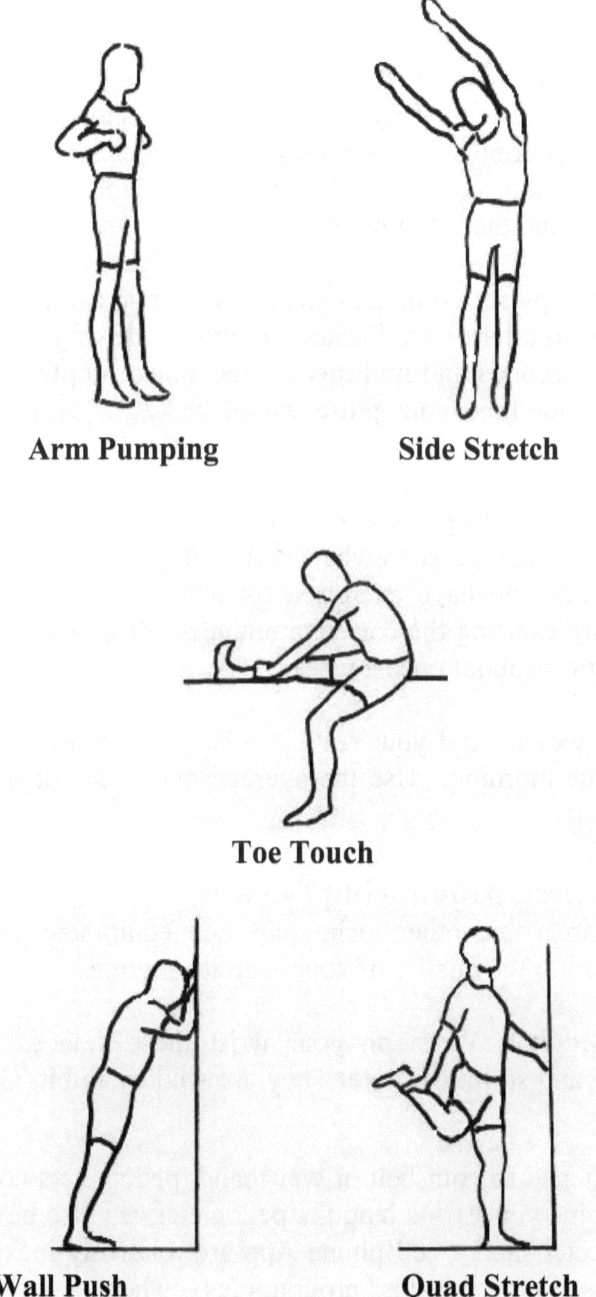

Figure 4.1: Stretching Exercises (c) to (g)
We are in the process of substituting female for the male figures.

Cool Down: A five to seven-minute cooling off period should follow an aerobic workout. During cool down keep moving, decrease your activity level slowly. End your workout with leg stretches such as toe touches, a wall push and a quad stretch.

Aerobic Exercise: Pulse Measurement

In order to monitor the intensity of exercise, you should stop during your workout and take your pulse immediately. This is because your pulse will fall quickly once you stop exercising. The trick is to find your pulse within a couple of seconds and then start counting.

Quickly place the tips of two fingers on one of the two carotid arteries in your neck. (Your carotid arteries are located on either side of your throat.) Count the beats for ten seconds and multiply by six. For example, if you count 20 beats in ten seconds then your pulse would be (20 x 6), or 120 beats per minute.

You are doing fine if your pulse is within your computed TTZ range. If your pulse is too slow, exercise somewhat harder; if your pulse is fast, exercise easier. Again, after you have exercised for some time you will be able to sense that you are exerting the correct amount of effort and need only check your exercising pulse about once a week.

(Note: The best way to find your resting pulse is to measure it immediately upon rising in the morning. Use the average over three days for the truest result.)

Aerobic Exercise: Monitoring Devices

The following are some other techniques and equipment you can use to measure and monitor the quality of your exercise regime.

Smart Watch Monitor: Worn on your wrist these devices measure your exercising pulse and so much more. They are sold by Fitbit, Garmin, Apple, Samsung, etc.

Pedometer: Fastened to your belt or waistband, pedometers count steps, and once you determine your stride length a pedometer can also be used to gauge distance. Pedometers and a cell phone App are relatively inexpensive. They are sometimes used in weight-loss programmes – where people are advised to accumulate at least 10,000 steps a day (which is equivalent to walking about seven kilometres).

<u>G.P.S. Monitor:</u> By determining your location, a Global Positioning System sensor can measure your speed, distance and pace during a workout.

<u>Power Meter:</u> Some cyclists use power meters to record power output, pedal revolutions, speed, time and distance. Most meters allow the data to be uploaded to a computer – but a power meter can be expensive.

Aerobic Exercise: Walking Programme

If your goal is to improve your general health and fitness, walking is a wonderful exercise. It is an exercise that you can do anywhere, that you can do outdoors or indoors, that requires no special equipment other than a good, comfortable pair of walking shoes, and that you can do well into your old age. Walking does have a downside. Because it is a relatively low-intensity exercise, to get a good workout you have to spend more time walking compared to most high-intensity exercises.

If you are more than 50 years old, or have been sedentary for some time, it is best to start with a walking routine that slowly but surely builds in intensity. If you walk hard enough, long enough and often enough, a walking workout can make you fit. A ten-week <u>beginner's routine</u> is shown in Table 4.4 on the following page.

The first session in week 1 starts with approximately three minutes of walking at an easy pace of about 4 km/hr. Continue your warm up with two minutes of stretching. (See the stretching exercises described on pages 47 and 48.) Then start walking more briskly, about 6 km/hr, but you should check your pulse and increase or decrease this to get your heart rate into a TTZ corresponding to about a 50 percent intensity level. After eight minutes, start your cool down by reducing your walking speed again to about 4 km/hr for three minutes. Conclude your session by doing about two minutes of stretching. The total workout time in week 1 is 18 minutes per session. The only part that changes in succeeding weeks (2 through 10), is the brisk walking portion of the workout continually increases from 8 minutes in week 1 to 30 minutes in week 10.

Week	Warm up Walking Minutes	Warm up Stretching (Minutes)	Brisk Walking Minutes	Cool Down Walking Minutes	Cool Down Stretching (Minutes)	Total Minutes per Session
1	3	2	8	3	2	18
2	3	2	10	3	2	20
3	3	2	12	3	2	22
4	3	2	14	3	2	24
5	3	2	16	3	2	26
6	3	2	18	3	2	28
7	3	2	20	3	2	30
8	3	2	23	3	2	33
9	3	2	26	3	2	36
10	3	2	30	3	2	40

Table 4.4: Walking Programme for Beginners

Walk at least three days a week for ten weeks. If you find a week particularly tiring, backup to the previous week (or repeat the week) before continuing with the programme. This is not a contest; you do not have to finish the programme in ten weeks. Once you complete the ten-week programme you can either stay on a walking routine, or go on to one of the more strenuous aerobic exercises.

If you decide to become a walker and want to improve, first go from walking three days per week to five days per week – at the same TTZ. To improve further gradually increase your total workout time from 40 to 60 minutes. To improve even more, gradually increase your walking speed, and TTZ, so that your exercise intensity level approaches 60 percent. Another good way to increase the intensity of your walking workout is to include some hills in your route. Incidentally, as you would expect, walking over hilly terrain also burns more calories than walking on level ground. On the two days you do not walk, try to get in 20 minutes of strengthening exercises (see page 55).

Because you will probably do most of your walking outside, you have to be aware of the weather forecast and have a backup plan for inclement weather. On bad-weather days, you could use an indoor walking site (like a mall, or an indoor track), walk on a treadmill, or do stretching or strength exercises instead of walking.

Aerobic Exercise: Jogging Programme

If you are in reasonably good condition, have completed the "Walking Programme for Beginners," or have been walking regularly, and have medical clearance, you can start a jogging programme. Table 4.5 (on the following page) illustrates a 13-week beginner's schedule. Try to get your pulse into your TTZ but don't overdue it. Gradually, over time, you want to increase both the intensity and distance of your jogging routine. However, if you don't have the physical makeup to do both, always choose endurance over intensity; i.e., choose distance rather than speed, choose to jog longer rather than faster.

The first session in week 1 starts with approximately five minutes of walking at an easy pace of about 4 km/hr. Continue your warm up with two minutes of stretching. (See the stretching exercises outlined on pages 47 and 48.) Then start walking more briskly, about 6 km/hr, but check your pulse and increase or decrease this to get your heart rate close to a TTZ that is roughly consistent with a 45 percent intensity level. After five minutes of brisk walking, jog for three minutes at a slightly higher heart rate, corresponding to about a 55 percent intensity level. Continue with another five minutes of brisk walking and a three-minute jog. Cool down by walking again but now at an easy speed of about 4 km/hr for three minutes. Conclude your session by doing about two minutes of stretching. The total workout time in week 1 is 26 minutes per session. In weeks 2 through 13, the time allotted to brisk walking decreases as the jogging time gradually increases.

Jog at least three days a week for 13 weeks. Again, if you find a week particularly tiring, backup to the previous week (or repeat the week) before continuing with the programme. Once you complete the programme, if you want to improve, first go from jogging three days per week to five days per week – at the same TTZ. To improve further gradually increase your total workout time from 30 to 60 minutes. On two of the days you do not jog, try to get in 20 minutes of strengthening exercises. To improve even more, gradually increase your jogging speed, and TTZ, so that your exercise intensity level approaches 65 percent. Another good way to increase the intensity of your jogging workout is to try to include some hills in your workout.

Week	Warm up (Minutes)		Brisk Walking & Jogging (Minutes)	Cool down (Minutes)		Total Minutes per Session
	Walk	Stretch		Walk	Stretch	
1	5	2	Walk 5 min, Jog 3 min Walk 5 min, Jog 3 min	3	2	26
2	5	2	Walk 4 min, Jog 5 min Walk 4 min, Jog 5 min	3	2	28
3	5	2	Walk 4 min, Jog 5 min Walk 4 min, Jog 5 min	3	2	28
4	5	2	Walk 4 min, Jog 6 min Walk 4 min, Jog 6 min	3	2	30
5	5	2	Walk 4 min, Jog 7min Walk 4 min, Jog 7 min	3	2	32
6	5	2	Walk 4 min, Jog 8 min Walk 4 min, Jog 8 min	3	2	34
7	5	2	Walk 4 min, Jog 9 min Walk 4 min, Jog 9 min	3	2	36
8	5	2	Walk 4 min, Jog 13 min Walk 4 min, Jog 13 min	3	2	27
9	5	2	Walk 4 min, Jog 15 min	3	2	29
10	5	2	Walk 4 min, Jog 17 min	3	2	31
11	5	2	Walk 2 min, Slow Jog 2 min then Jog 17 min	3	2	33
12	5	2	Walk 2 min, Slow Jog 3 min then Jog 17 min	3	2	34
13	5	2	Slow Jog 5 min then Jog 17 min	3	2	34

Table 4.5: Jogging Programme for Beginners

Because you will undoubtedly do most of your jogging outside, you have to be aware of the weather forecast and have a contingency plan for inclement weather. On bad-weather days, you might use an indoor track, try an alternate

exercise like jogging on a treadmill, or do stretching or strength exercises.
As always, stop exercising immediately if you experience tightness or pain in your chest, become light-headed or dizzy, are severely breathless, lose muscle control or are nauseous. These are warning signs of over exertion and you definitely should lower your exercise-intensity level. If you experience these symptoms, it is also a good idea to seek medical attention.

Be aware that the pounding your body gets from jogging usually takes its toll over time. Many joggers have recurring, nagging injuries, particularly to their legs and feet. If you begin to suffer chronic injuries, remember there are other high-intensity aerobic exercises for which your body might be better suited. At that point, you might consider switching to cycling, a rowing machine, etcetera. Before abandoning jogging altogether, however, you might want to cut back, and only jog two days per week and try another high-intensity non-impact exercise the other three days of the week. Variety will also make your workout more enjoyable.

Your Body's Muscles

Your body has approximately 650 muscles that account for more than half your body weight. (You also have about 206 bones.) Figures 4.3 and 4.4, on the following pages, show the location of 17 of the muscles you will most likely hear trainers and health club members talking about as you workout. Many of these muscles are also referred to in the "Strength Programmes" section that follows immediately. If you want to know more about your musculature, pick up a Human Anatomy and Physiology text at your local library.

Strength-Building Programmes

As good as aerobic exercises are, they contribute little to building upper-body strength. If you are a beginner interested in strength training it is probably worthwhile to start by joining a health club, where you can get professional instruction on the proper use of exercise equipment, from dumbbells to rowing machines, and where you can compare different exercise routines. Another possibility is to hire a personal trainer for a couple of sessions to get you started on a programme personalized to your fitness level and to teach you correct exercise techniques.

Of all the many strengthening options available, I personally prefer free weights (actually dumbbells) because they can be used at home. Working out at home has some significant advantages. First, your workout takes less time

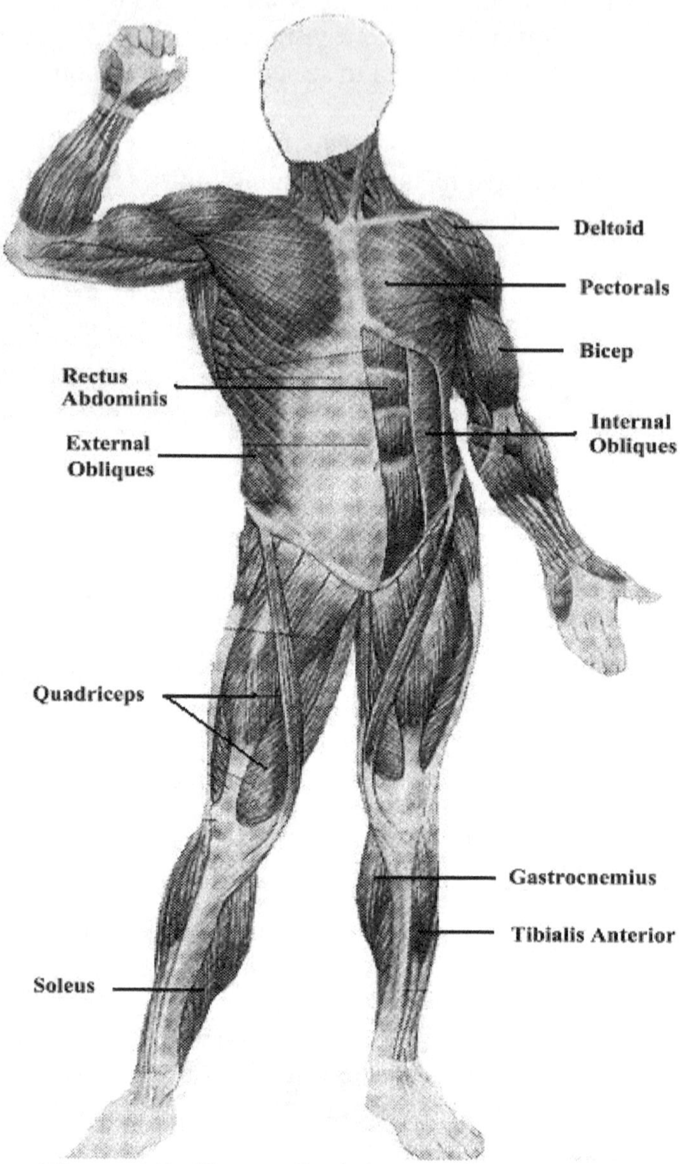

Figure 4.2: Human Body's Muscles – Front View

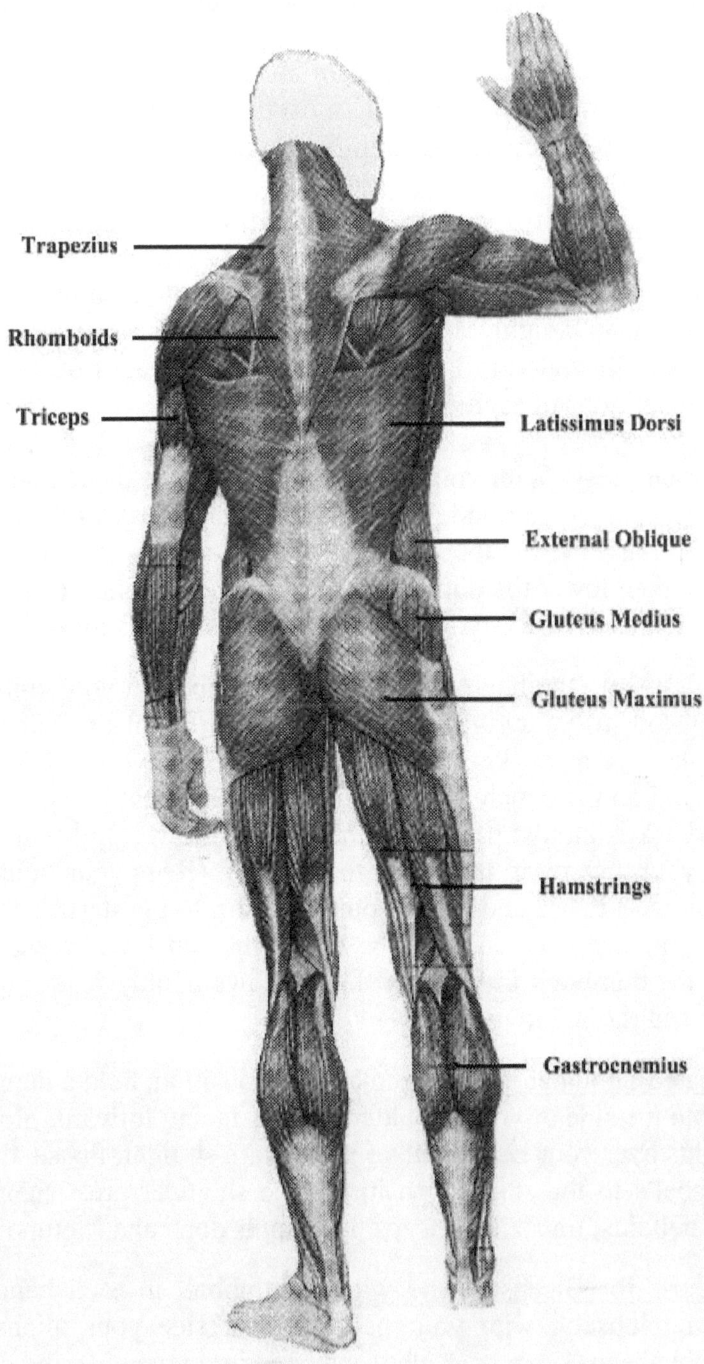

Figure 4.3: Human Body's Muscles – Rear View

The seven dumbbell exercises that follow comprise a total-body workout, suitable for beginners, that involve all the major muscle groups. When done consecutively without stopping a series of exercises is called a circuit. To start, use the same dumbbell weight for all the exercises, a weight that allows you to do 10 to 15 repetitions of the most difficult exercise in the circuit. For the first week do one circuit per training session.

Your goal should be two circuits per session, which should take you about 20 minutes (with a two to three-minute rest between circuits). When you are comfortable at this level you are ready to increase the dumbbell weight – but by no more than roughly 10 percent (or one pound minimum). The seven exercises are illustrated in Figures 4.4 and 4.5 on pages 60 and 61. Perform 10 to 15 repetitions of each exercise.

a) <u>Bench Press</u>: With your head and back on the bench, hold a dumbbell in each hand to the side of your shoulders, palms facing each other. Slowly raise the dumbbells extending your arms above your shoulders. Pause, then lower the dumbbells down to the starting position. The bench press primarily works your pectorals, triceps and deltoids.

b) <u>One–Arm Dumbbell Row</u>: Hold a dumbbell in your right hand, palm facing toward your right thigh. Stand to the right of your weight bench and place your left knee on the bench. Support yourself by putting your left hand on the bench. (Flex your right knee slightly and lean forward so your back is almost parallel to the floor.) Slowly pull your right arm up until your upper arm is parallel to the floor. (Keep your right arm close to your torso.) Pause and lower your right arm to the starting position. After you complete a set, stand to the left of the bench and repeat the exercise with the dumbbell in your left hand. Rows mainly work your latissimus dorsi and rhomboid muscles.

c) <u>Seated Shoulder Press</u>: From a seated position, hold a dumbbell in each hand to the side of your shoulders, palms facing forward. Slowly raise the weights over your head until your arms are straight. Pause, then lower the dumbbells to the starting position. The shoulder press mainly exercises your deltoids, trapezius, triceps, latissimus dorsi and rhomboid muscles.

c) <u>Curls for Biceps</u>: Stand with a dumbbell in each hand, your arms hanging loosely, with your palms to the side your thighs and facing straight ahead. Keep your elbows tucked into your side and slowly lift the dumbbells until they are approximately shoulder high. Pause and lower the dumbbells to the starting position. Curls chiefly work your biceps.

e) <u>Tricep Extension</u>: With a dumbbell in your right hand, assume the same initial position as in the one-arm dumbbell row. Slowly move your right arm rearward until it is nearly parallel to the floor. Pause and then return the dumbbell to the starting position without bending your arm. After completing a set, stand to the left of the bench and repeat the exercise with the dumbbell in your left hand. This exercise mainly works your triceps.

f) <u>Front Squats</u>: Stand with a dumbbell in each hand, to the side of your shoulders, palms facing each other (inward). Slowly bend your knees and lower your body until your thighs are almost parallel to the floor. Try to keep your heels on the floor. Pause and gradually raise your body by straightening your knees. Squats work your gluteus, quadriceps and hamstrings.

g) <u>Curls for Abs</u>: This is not a weight lifting exercise but is a useful part of any routine. Lie face up on a floor mat with your hands folded over your chest and your legs bent. Keeping your feet flat on the mat, slowly curl your torso up and toward your thighs until your shoulder blades are off the mat. Pause, then return to the starting position. This exercise works your rectus abdominis muscles – your abs.

Remember to do about five minutes of aerobic and stretching exercises before and after your strength exercises, and to workout two to three (non-consecutive) days per week. Why non-consecutive days? Because strengthening exercises work a muscle until it's fatigued, and a day off is needed for muscles to recover, repair and rebuild. And remember to listen to your body to determine your level of exertion. Don't over do it!

A final word about breathing properly: Never hold your breath during weight training. This can cause your blood pressure to get dangerously high. Rather, breathe naturally and try to exhale during a lift.

Additional Strengthening Exercises

As your conditioning improves, you may want a more challenging workout. This can be accomplished in a number of ways. One method is to use two pairs of variable weight dumbbells, with a different weight loaded on each set of dumbbells. Now, you can more closely equalize the difficulty of the different exercises by using the lighter pair for harder exercises and the heavier pair of dumbbells for easier exercises. Yet another way to make your workout more demanding is to add one or more of the following exercises to your routine:

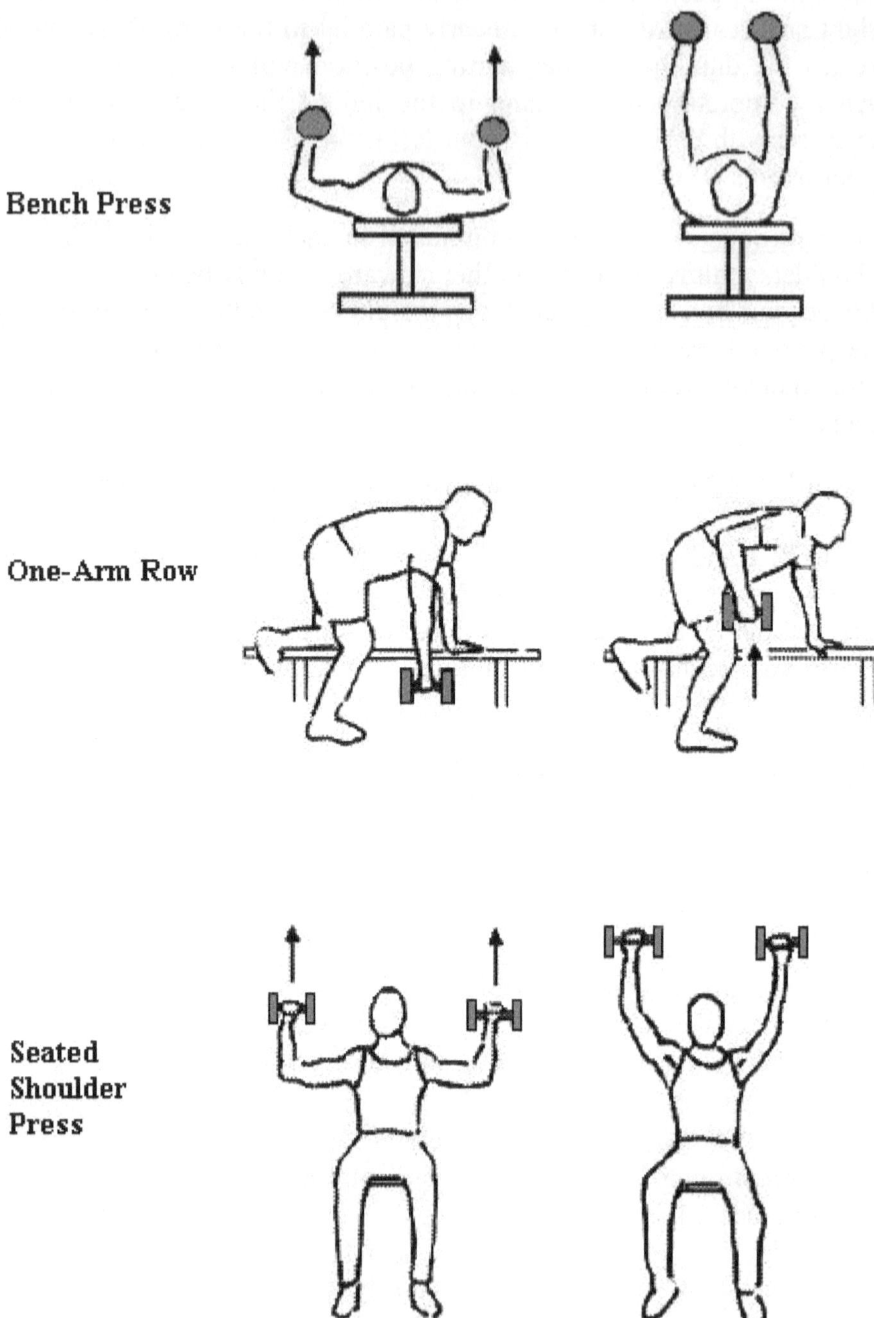

Figure 4.4: Strengthening Exercises (a) to (c)
We are in the process of substituting female for the male figures.

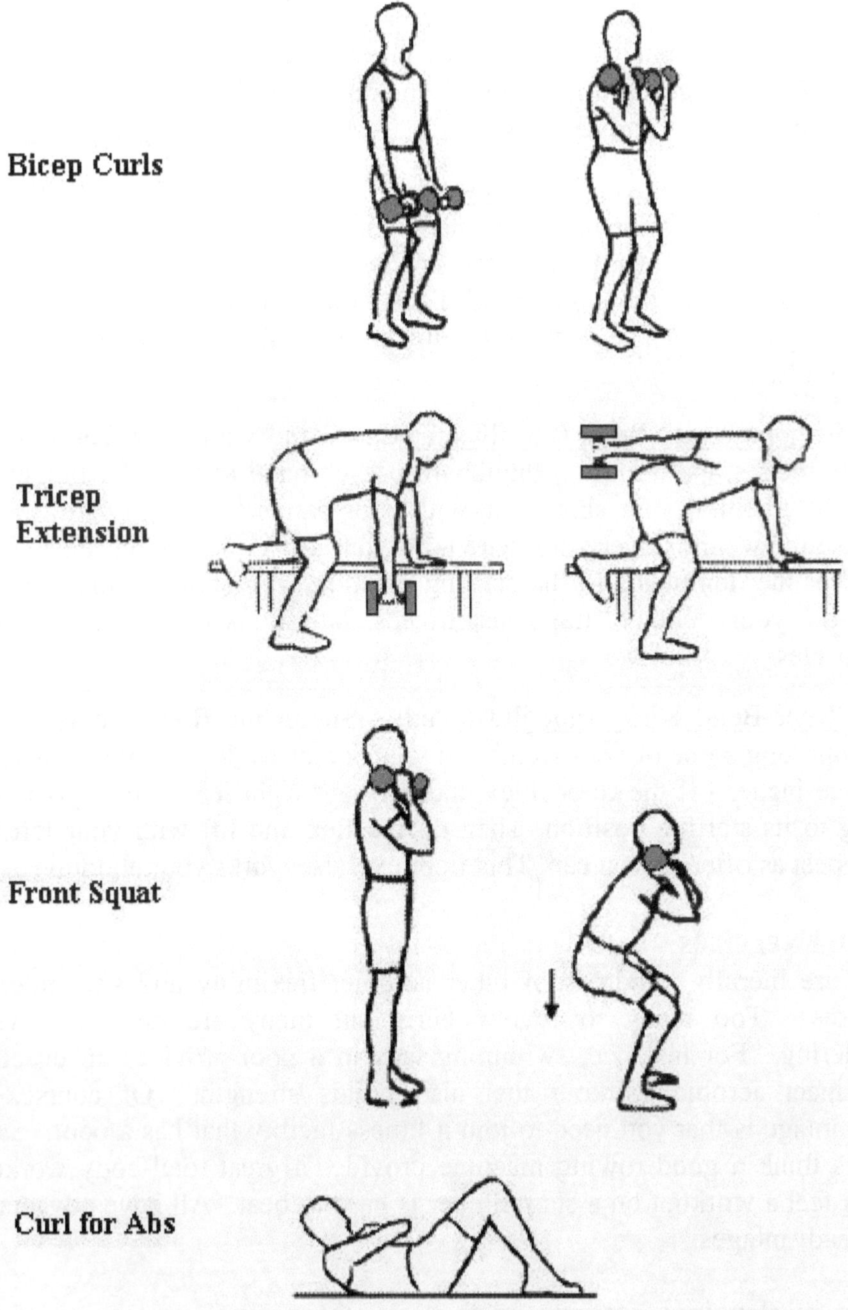

Figure 4.5: Strengthening Exercises (d to g)
We are in the process of substituting female for the male figures.

h) <u>Dumbbell Fly (not illustrated)</u>: With your head and back on a bench, hold a dumbbell in each hand and fully extend your arms upward with your palms facing each other. Keeping your arms fully extended, slowly lower the dumbbells sideways to chest level. Pause, then return the dumbbells to the starting position. The dumbbell fly primarily trains your pectorals, triceps and deltoids.

i) <u>Dumbbell Pullover (not illustrated)</u>: With your head and back on a bench, hold a dumbbell in each hand and fully extend your arms upward with your palms facing each other. Allow your arms to bend as you lower the dumbbells behind your head. Pause, then return the dumbbells to the starting position. The dumbbell pullover primarily works your triceps and deltoids.

j) <u>Standing Back Press (not illustrated)</u>: Stand with your feet about 30 centimetres apart. Hold a dumbbell in each hand at shoulder height and slightly behind your shoulders, with your palms facing forward. Slowly raise the weights over your head until your arms are straight. Pause, then lower the dumbbells to the starting position. The shoulder press mainly works your deltoids, trapezius, triceps, latissimus dorsi and rhomboid muscles.

k) <u>Knee-Bend Kicks (not illustrated)</u>: Sit on the floor and lean back supporting some of your weight on your forearms. Raise both heals about three inches off the floor. Flex and lift your right leg. Return your right leg to its starting position. Then do the flex and lift with your left leg. Repeat as often as you can. This floor exercise works your abdominals.

Other Exercises

There are literally hundreds of other aerobic, flexibility and strengthening exercises. Too many to review here, but many are definitely worth considering. For instance, swimming laps in a pool provides an excellent low-impact aerobic workout that also builds strength. Of course, the disadvantage is that you need to join a fitness facility that has a pool. Some trainers think a good rowing machine provides a great total-body workout. Others feel a workout on a stairclimber is hard to beat. All have advantages and disadvantages.

In fact, most trainers recommend that you change your routine every few months to add variety. Some advocate alternating exercises every other session. For example, if you jog and lift weights on alternate days, you avoid repeating movements on consecutive days. As bonus, you will also most likely avoid the injuries that are often associated with day-after-day repetitive motion.

Missed Workouts

Inevitably, you will miss some workouts. It may be due to a heavy work schedule, a minor illness, or an injury. If you are injured or ill, wait for the injury to heal, or for when you feel like your normal self before resuming your exercise routine.

If you miss only a day or two, you can undoubtedly just pick up where you left off as if nothing happened. If you miss a week or more, however, you will probably have lost some of your fitness gains and might have to resume at a somewhat lower exercising-intensity level. This means that when you come back after missing some aerobic sessions, you might have to exercise at a slightly lower TTZ, or shorten the duration of your workout. And when you return after missing some strengthening sessions, you might want to reduce the weight you are lifting or reduce the number of repetitions.

Incidentally, physical fitness can be maintained only by regular workouts. If your exercise frequency drops to one day a week, half your fitness gains will be lost in 10 weeks. If exercise is stopped completely, virtually all your accumulated fitness benefits will be lost in five weeks! Therefore, if you want to keep that state of well-being, feeling better, looking better, it is important to make regular aerobic exercise part of your lifestyle.

Exercising in Hot Weather

When you engage in vigorous exercise, your body generates a great deal of heat, and your body temperature can rise from 37°C up to 38.5°C. (A body temperature of 40.5°C is life threatening.)

High ambient temperatures and high humidity are a concern because both influence how effectively you transfer the heat you generate to the environment. High ambient temperatures are an obvious cooling problem, but high levels of humidity also cause cooling difficulties by hindering the evaporation of perspiration. As a result, on days when it is both hot and humid it is even more difficult to transfer heat from your body to the surrounding ambient air. This combination can cause your body temperature to rise to dangerous levels. **On hot humid summer days, therefore, you must guard against overdoing it**.

Heat Index: Adopted by the U.S. National Weather Service, the heat index, or apparent temperature, combines the effects of air (dry bulb) temperature and relative humidity. (Heat index values are expressed in either degrees Celsius or Fahrenheit.) The heat index is not perfect but it is considered the best available guide for the general population. As expected, Table 4.6 shows that when the heat index rises, so do health risks. In hot weather, the major threats are heat stroke, heat exhaustion and dehydration.

Category	Heat Index		Heat-Related Risks
	(°F)	(°C)	
Caution	80 to 90°F	27 to 32°C	Unexpected fatigue possible with prolonged exposure and/or physical activity.
Extreme Caution	90 to 105°F	32 to 41°C	Muscle cramps and/or heat exhaustion possible with prolonged exposure and/or physical activity.
Danger	105 to 129°F	41 to 54°C	Muscle cramps and/or heat exhaustion likely. Heat stroke possible with long exposure and/or physical activity.
Extreme Danger	130°F or higher	54°C or higher	Heat stroke likely.

Table 4.6: Health Risks vs. Hot Weather Conditions (Heat Index)

Heat Exhaustion: As described in Table 4.6, when heat index values reach 32 to 41°C, you could suffer muscle cramps, particularly in your legs and heat exhaustion. The symptoms of heat exhaustion are pale clammy skin, dizziness or fainting, a rapid pulse, fast breathing, and nausea. If you experience any of these problems, get to a cool place, lie down and sip water. You may also need to seek medical attention.

Heat Stroke: Much more dangerous is heat stroke, which results when extremely hot weather triggers a malfunction of the body's thermostat, causing the body temperature to rise to 40°C or higher. Symptoms of heat stroke are confusion or loss of consciousness, flushed, hot and dry skin, a strong and rapid pulse. **Heat stroke is a medical emergency**. Move the person to the coolest accessible place and call your local emergency phone number. Some first aid measures include removing some of the person's clothing and sponging with cool water.

Dehydration: Everyone knows drinking water is important for good health, but it is even more important on hot days while you are exercising. During vigorous exercise, you can lose one to two litres of water per hour in sweat, so it is essential to use common sense and stay hydrated. And in hot weather, drink plenty of water and fruit juice even if you do not feel thirsty.

Relative Humidity (%)	Air Temperature (°C)											
	28	30	32	34	36	38	40	42	44	46	48	50
10	27	28	30	32	33	35	37	39	41	43	45	48
15	27	28	30	32	34	36	38	41	43	46	49	52
20	27	28	30	32	34	37	39	42	46	49	53	57
25	27	28	30	33	35	38	41	45	48	53	57	62
30	27	29	31	33	36	39	43	47	52	57	62	
35	27	29	32	34	38	41	46	50	56	61		
40	28	30	32	35	39	43	48	54	60	66		
45	28	30	33	37	41	46	51	58	64			
50	28	31	34	38	43	49	55	62				
55	29	32	36	40	46	52	59	66				
60	30	33	37	42	48	55	63					
65	30	34	39	44	51	59	67					
70	31	35	40	47	54	63						
75	31	36	42	49	58	67						
80	32	38	44	52	61							
85	33	39	47	55	65							
90	34	41	49	58								
95	35	42	52	62								
100	36	44	54									

Note: Exposure to full sun can increase heat index by 8°C.

Table 4.7: Heat Index for Various Temperature-Humidity Combinations

Yet another annoying problem in hot weather is chafing. Skin irritation can happen anywhere clothing touches your skin. If you are bothered by this troubling condition try different clothing styles, fabrics, or simply coat the affected area with petroleum jelly.

Before exercising outdoors in hot weather, check your latest local weather forecast. If the forecast does not incorporate the heat index, you can use the forecasted air temperature and relative humidity to determine a heat index value using Table 4.7. (Note the heat index values in Table 4.7 are in degrees Celsius and the colours in the table correspond to those in the risk categories shown in Table 4.6.)

Frankly, unless you are relatively young and in very good physical condition, **it is not a good idea to engage in vigorous outdoor exercise when the heat index is over 33°C**. Despite this advice, if you persist on exercising on very hot days, make sure you wear loose-fitting, light-collared clothes; avoid the blazing sun (which can increase the heat index by 8°C) by working out early in the morning or the evening; wear a hat and use sun screen; reduce the intensity of your workout; and drink plenty of water. In addition, be aware that the temperature of paved roadways can easily exceed 38°C even when the ambient air temperature is only 26°C. Therefore, if you are intent on jogging on hot days it is best to do so in a shaded park. Finally when you workout in very hot weather always let someone know when and where you will be exercising and what time you plan to return.

Exercising in Cold Weather

The ideal exercise temperature range is about 4 to 29°C with a wind speed less than 25 kph, but many people continue to exercise outdoors at temperatures well below 4°C. Generally, cold weather is less dangerous to an exerciser – but definitely not risk-free. When you exercise outdoors in cold weather you encounter an entirely new set of difficulties. Besides often-treacherous footing on snow-covered or icy surfaces, you must contend with low temperatures and the wind.

Wind Chill Temperature Index: Basic physics states that when heat leaves an object the temperature of the object drops. The same principle applies to your body. As heat leaves your body, your temperature drops and you feel cold. Very low ambient temperatures combined with the wind increase the amount of heat leaving your body. As the wind speed increases, the temperature of any exposed skin drops even further. The Wind Chill Temperature Index was developed in an effort to quantify this phenomenon, and is a measure of the relative discomfort due to combined cold temperature and wind. In essence, the wind-chill temperature lets you know what the outside air temperature "feels like," based on the heat loss from skin exposed to low air temperatures and the wind.

In 2001, the U.S. National Weather Service and Environment Canada jointly issued a new Wind Chill Temperature Index. Table 4.8 presents a version of the Wind Chill Temperature Index issued by the U.S. National Weather Service. (The wind-chill temperatures in Table 4.8 are in degrees Celsius and the colours in the table correspond to those in the risk categories shown in Table 4.9. Note that exposure to bright sunshine helps, because the sun may increase wind-chill temperatures by 5 to 10°C. The combination of low air temperatures and increasing wind speeds can result in incredibly low wind-chill temperatures. For instance, Table 4.8 shows that an air temperature of -34°C and a wind speed of 60 kph produces a wind chill temperature of -56°C. Now that's cold! And dangerous!

One of the **potential consequences of very low wind chill temperatures is frostbite**. Table 4.9 (on page 69) employs the Canadian interpretation of frostbite risks rather than the U.S. version. (After all, who knows more about cold weather than Canadians?) **Other serious cold weather related conditions are hypothermia and heart attack.**

Frostbite: When body tissue freezes the injury is called frostbite, which usually strikes fingers, toes, nose and ears. Frostbitten skin is numb, hard and pale, and requires immediate medical attention. If you suspect you have frostbite, get indoors as quickly as you can and call or send for help. First aid steps include covering the frozen area with a blanket and drinking a warm non-alcoholic beverage.

Hypothermia: Prolonged exposure to extreme cold, especially during exercise, can result in a depletion of energy stores (calories) which can cause a drop in body temperature. This in turn can cause a gradual mental slowing. The stricken person becomes increasingly unreasonable, clumsy, irritable, sleepy, and eventually lapses into a coma. This is a life-threatening condition. (Severe hypothermia can lead to cardiac and respiratory failure and death.) To help, your first move should be to call your local emergency phone number for help. Then start first aid (which is beyond the scope of this book).

Heart Attack: As the air temperature drops, your body's air-warming system may not be able to adequately heat the cold air entering your mouth and flowing down your windpipe. As a result, the incoming cold air may cause your coronary arteries to constrict – resulting in a heart attack – particularly if you are not in good condition.

Air Temp (°C)	Wind Speed (kph)										
	0	10	20	30	40	50	60	70	80	90	100
4	4	2	0	-1	-2	-3	-3	-4	-4	-5	-5
2	2	-1	-3	-4	-5	-5	-6	-7	-7	-7	-8
0	0	-3	-5	-7	-7	-8	-9	-9	-10	-10	-11
-2	-2	-6	-8	-9	-10	-11	-12	-12	-13	-13	-14
-4	-4	-8	-10	-12	-13	-14	-14	-15	-16	-16	-16
-6	-6	-11	-13	-14	-15	-16	-17	-18	-18	-19	-19
-8	-8	-13	-15	-17	-18	-19	-20	-21	-21	-22	-22
-10	-10	-15	-18	-20	-21	-22	-23	-23	-24	-25	-25
-12	-12	-18	-20	-22	-23	-25	-25	-26	-27	-27	-28
-14	-14	-20	-23	-25	-26	-27	-28	-29	-30	-30	-31
-16	-16	-22	-25	-27	-29	-30	-31	-32	-33	-33	-34
-18	-18	-25	-28	-30	-31	-33	-34	-35	-35	-36	-37
-20	-20	-27	-30	-33	-34	-35	-36	-37	-38	-39	-40
-22	-22	-30	-33	-35	-37	-38	-39	-40	-41	-42	-43
-24	-24	-32	-36	-38	-39	-41	-42	-43	-44	-45	-45
-26	-26	-34	-38	-40	-42	-44	-45	-46	-47	-48	-48
-28	-28	-37	-41	-43	-45	-46	-48	-49	-50	-50	-51
-30	-30	-39	-43	-46	-48	-49	-50	-51	-52	-53	-54
-32	-32	-42	-46	-48	-50	-52	-53	-54	-55	-56	-57
-34	-34	-44	-48	-51	-53	-54	-56	-57	-58	-59	-60
-36	-36	-46	-51	-53	-56	-57	-59	-60	-61	-62	-63
-38	-38	-49	-53	-56	-58	-60	-61	-63	-64	-65	-66
-40	-40	-51	-56	-59	-61	-63	-64	-65	-67	-68	-69

Table 4.8: Wind-Chill Temperature vs. Air Temperature & Wind Speed

Wind Chill Temperature	Frostbite Risk for Most People	Exposure Time
4°C to -27°C	Low	---
-28°C to -37°C	Medium	10 to 30 minutes
-37°C to -47°C	High	5 to 10 minutes
-48°C to -53°C	Higher	2 to 5 minutes
-54°C to -67°C	Highest	2 minutes or less

Table 4.9: Frostbite Risk vs. Wind-Chill Temperature

At a wind chill temperature of approximately -28°C the risk of frostbite starts to increase. Unless you are skiing cross-country or downhill, or engaged in another winter sport that requires you to be outdoors, in bitterly-cold weather, the best advice is to exercise indoors. Furthermore, it is **not a good idea to exercise outdoors when the wind-chill temperature is below -30°C**. At this wind chill temperature any exposed skin will freeze in about 20 minutes. In brief then, even if you are relatively young and in very good condition, rather than exercising outdoors in very cold weather, consider joining a health club, setting up a small workout space at your home, or walking in an enclosed mall.

Upshot of Cold Weather: Once the wind-chill temperature reaches approximately -12°C exercising outdoors becomes increasingly uncomfortable. Even if you are an outdoor enthusiast, at this wind chill you may want to think about changing to an indoor exercise routine until the weather moderates.

Dressing for Cold Weather: Notwithstanding our best advice, if you still intend to exercise outdoors in frigid weather, wear layers of loose-fitting, lightweight, warm clothing. The layer closest to your skin should be a thin layer of a synthetic wicking material that draws perspiration away from your body. The second layer should provide insulation. Water-resistant fleece is a good option. Your third, outer layer, should be windproof and waterproof with a hood. Generally, mittens are warmer than gloves, and wool or polypropylene socks insulate and wick moisture. Wear a head sock that covers your entire head and neck with openings only for breathing and vision. Consider covering your mouth with a scarf to cause the air you breathe to be slightly warmer and more humid. Further, wear goggles or wrap-around sunglasses to protect your eyes from wind and ultraviolet radiation. And make sure to stay dry.

In addition, remember to drink plenty of water – even in cold weather – to make up for water you lose when you sweat during strenuous exercise.

Exercise Risks and Problems

Certain situations may occur that indicate you may be doing too much, exercising too hard. For example, regardless of your pulse rate you should never be left completely breathless by your aerobic exercise. A good rule to remember is: **You are exercising too hard if you cannot carry on a conversation while you are jogging, cycling, etcetera**. A feeling of having worked hard is fine, sweating is good, but not a feeling of undo fatigue.

Perhaps the most frequent problems faced by exercisers are injuries of the joints and muscles: sprains and strains, knee pain, elbow pain, back pain, neck pain, shin splints and stress fractures. Most happen when you exercise too hard. Potentially serious problems are signalled if you experience any of the following symptoms during or after exercise. The symptoms include but are not limited to any abnormal heart action such as an irregular heart rhythm; pain or pressure in the middle of your chest; pain in an arm or your neck; dizziness, fainting or light-headedness; severe exhaustion; sudden loss of coordination; or confusion. If any of these symptoms are experienced, stop exercising immediately and get medical help.

Avoiding Injury

My good retired friend and workout partner Dr. Kanaar's specialty was rehabilitation medicine but he also preached what he called "preventive medicine," that is avoiding injury by practicing a common-sense approach to exercise:

- **Have a medical check-up and then set realistic fitness goals.**

- **Build up your exercise intensity gradually over many weeks, months.**

- **After you eat a meal, wait two hours before exercising.**

- **Buy good shoes and equipment that are suitable for your exercise routine.**

- **Use safety and protective equipment when appropriate, such as helmet when you bicycle, and goggles when you play handball, squash or racquetball.**

- **On hot days, follow the precautions in the section "Exercising in Hot Weather."**

- **On cold days, follow the precautions in the section "Exercising in Cold Weather."**

- **If you insist on working out in very hot or cold weather, always let someone know when and where you will be exercising and when you are planning to return.**

- **If you are new to a gym or health club, attend an orientation session before you use any unfamiliar exercise equipment. Otherwise, read the operating instructions carefully and ask someone qualified to help you.**

- **For aerobic activities, warm up slowly to reach your TTZ and cool down slowly after you exercise.**

- **Do not increase the difficulty of any activity (e.g., your walking or jogging distance, the amount of weight you lift) by more than 10 percent per week.**

- **Jog on softer surfaces such as a level grass field, a dirt path, or a running track.**

- **After exercising wait 30 minutes before eating.**

- **As a final point, if you experience some early warning pain stop exercising.**

Many minor leg injuries of the muscles and joints can be easily treated using the well-known R.I.C.E. method, i.e., rest, ice, compression, elevation.

Rest. You may not have to avoid all physical activity; just taking it easy might be fine.

Ice. Apply ice for 15 minutes several times a day for as long as there is any swelling.

Compress the area with a bandage or sleeve to help control swelling.

Elevate the injured area above the level of your heart.

On the other hand, if early pain is ignored and you continue exercising, a minor injury may become more serious.

Keep an Exercise Log

Individuals who keep a record of their exercise generally exercise more often and have more success over the long term. How should you go about this? Keep an exercise log. A sample Daily Exercise Log is shown in Table 4.10 with two days filled in.

Day	Aerobic Exercise	Distance	Time	Heart Rate	Strength Exercise	Weight	Reps	Sets
Mon 07/10	Walking	6.5 km	65 min	124	None			
Tues 07/11	Walking	6.75 km	72 min	122	Bench Press	5 kg	12	2
					Rows	8 kg	12	2
					Tricep Extensio	5 kg	12	2
					Press	8 kg	12	2
					Curls	8 kg	12	2
					Squats	8 kg	10	1
					Abs	N/A	25	2

Table 4.10: Sample Exercise Log

A Fitness Expert's Ideal Exercise

A prominent 43-year-old professor of physiology was asked at the end of a speech to a group of business executives to give her definition of the "ideal" exercise. Without hesitation she reeled off her checklist, saying her ideal exercise would be one which:

- Is aerobic, preferably where the arms as well as the legs are used.
- Is efficient, yielding the maximum fitness return for the minimum time investment.
- Can be done every day if desired, outside or indoors, i.e., is not weather dependent.
- Does not require any special equipment or facilities.
- Requires only one participant.
- It's fun!

She went on to tell of her extremely busy schedule: laboratory research, classroom teaching, speaking engagements, consulting. Yet she said she exercised every day virtually without fail, whether teaching in Chicago, visiting her publisher in New York City, or speaking in St. Louis. She bragged that her total time expenditure on overt exercise was usually only 40 minutes a day.

Then she described the exercise programme she now follows that she felt most closely met her ideal. She said she was a "morning person" and that she got in her daily exercise first thing in the morning. She warmed up by doing stretching exercises for a few minutes, and then while watching the morning news on television she jogged in place for 30 minutes - making sure her pulse reached approximately 145 beats per minute - high enough to put her at the 70% exercise intensity level. She did a few sets of press-ups, abdominal curls and finally more stretching as she cooled off. Then still perspiring she jumped into the shower, she would have taken anyway, towelled off and was ready for breakfast. She added that when she was home she also jogged in place, and for variety every other day she rode a stationary bike. She exercised every day.

In conclusion, she admitted that her real passion was tennis which she played whenever she could, but which she said was only an adjunct to her exercise programme not the backbone. Her reason: She could not reasonably expect to fit at least three or four tennis workouts a week into her schedule. Arranging for courts and partners, driving to the tennis courts, changing clothes, taking a needed extra shower, the entire process took more than two hours per session. Besides, a good deal of the time she missed her tennis match because she was out of town or too busy to take the time!

My Personal Exercise Routine

I started jogging in the late 1960's. Of course I was much younger then. I jogged five to eight kilometres almost every morning and worked out with free weights (dumbbells) on the days I didn't jog. After 20 years of jogging, the constant pounding resulted in a troubling number of chronic minor leg and foot injuries. So I switched to walking and I have been walking ever since. Now I'm a semi-retired senior citizen; so I have more time than most. For the past 15 years, from 6:00 to 7:00 am, I take a brisk walk covering about 6.5 kilometres. Most days I walk outside but when the weather is bad I head for a nearby enclosed shopping mall. For variety, every other day, I power walk in place for about 40 minutes using one of my six exercise DVDs to set the rhythm; then I complete my workout doing two circuits of the dumbbell exercises described starting on page 60.

In warmer weather I golf (walk 18 holes) or hike (about eight miles) two or three times a week. On those days - that's my workout. Although just a week before this writing, I finished my brisk one-hour morning walk followed by 20 minutes of dumbbell exercises. Then later in the day a friend called and next thing I know I'm playing 18 holes of golf. Walking – of course. In total, I exercised 5 hours and 45 minutes, burned about 2000 Calories, and felt strong, definitely not tired, at the end of the day. Not bad for a senior!

In summary, one day I walk outside for an hour; the following day I power walk in place for 40 minutes using an exercise DVD and also lift weights; the next day I'm back to walking outside. I've been doing this for 15 years. I exercise every day without fail. Every day! And because walking is the central part of my programme, I almost never suffer an exercise-related injury.

My exercise routine combined with a sensible diet have kept me trim over the years (within three pounds of my college-graduation weight). Most people think I'm younger than my chronological age – and I feel great!

Workout to Feel Good & Stay Healthy

If your goal is a chiselled body with washboard abs and the endurance and strength of a triathlon athlete, you're reading the wrong book. Sure the aerobic and strength routines outlined here will help you get in shape, slim down a bit and get somewhat stronger - but your body is not going to be transformed into the physique of a world-class athlete.

This chapter is about how you should workout to get fit so that you feel good and stay healthy. And you're not going to get fit just because you join a fancy health club with lots of high-tech equipment - if you only workout once or twice a week, every other week. Joining a health club is great, if you use it – consistently.

The words that describe our kind of workout are consistent, determined, steady, persistent, dogged, unswerving, gritty, single-minded. Get the point? In our kind of workout, you decide that you will workout at least five days a week; that an aerobic exercise will form the core of your workout, and that you will incorporate some strengthening exercises two days a week. After that, it doesn't matter exactly what exercises you choose, what equipment you use, or what facility you use. These are secondary factors. What matters most is that you exercise consistently. **To improve muscle tone and overall fitness, feel good and stay healthy, you should exercise at least five days per week, day after day, week after week, year after year – for as long as you are physically able.** Remember the key words: consistent, determined, steady, persistent, dogged, unswerving, gritty, single-minded. Consistent!

Of course, there's a bit more involved. To feel good and stay healthy, you must also eat properly. That's next in Chapter 5 - Nutrition Basics.

5. NUTRITION BASICS

In the opinion of many researchers the makeup of the diet eaten by the majority of people in most industrialized countries is the single most important factor, albeit not the only one, accounting for the high incidence of death from coronary heart disease and stroke. It is no coincidence that accompanying the high mortality numbers is an increase in the amount of fat we eat, an increase in the number of calories consumed per capita, and the inevitable increase in the average weight of our citizens. All are directly attributable to our diet.

Healthy eating habits, the result of sensible nutritional practices, must be an integral part of any physical fitness programme. In this chapter you will learn how to improve the "nutritional quality" of the food you eat, and, as expected, we will also point out foods that you should avoid, i.e., those foods that are loaded with "nutritionally-empty calories."

Metabolic Pathways

Early men and women evolved a storage system for survival during alternating periods of plenty and fasting. Physiologists describe these two functional periods as the absorptive state, when the food we eat enters the blood and lymph from the gastrointestinal tract (GI tract), and the post-absorptive stage, or fasting state, when the GI tract is empty and energy is supplied by the body's energy storage system – the body's adipose tissue, or fat.

During the absorptive period diagrammed in Figure 5.1 (on page 77), fat droplets (triglycerides) are absorbed directly into the lymph and stored in the adipose tissue. Carbohydrates (primarily in the form of glucose) and protein (amino acids) enter the blood stream. All the blood leaving the GI tract goes to the liver.

Although glucose is the body's major energy source during the absorptive state, much of the glucose is converted in the liver to glycogen and stored as an immediately available energy source. A small fraction, of the amino acids in the food you eat, is used for energy; another fraction is used to resynthesize continuously degrading body tissue. Any excess calories, whether carbohydrate, protein, or fat, are stored in the adipose tissue as fat.

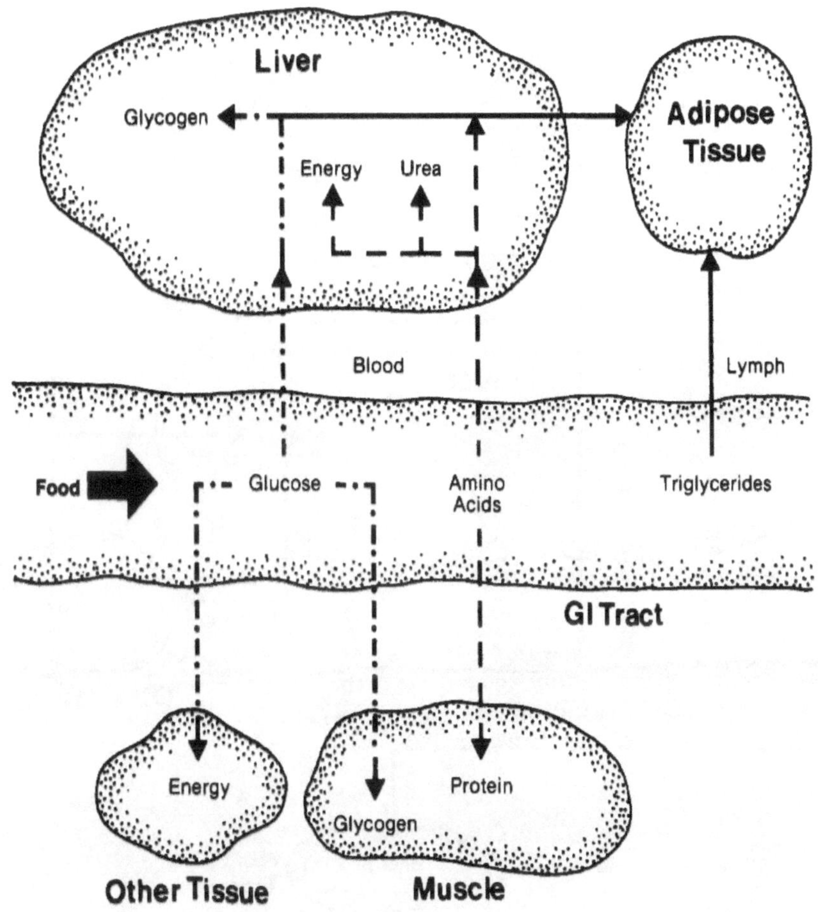

Figure 5.1: Metabolic Pathways - Absorptive Stage

During the post-absorptive period illustrated in Figure 5.2 (on page 78), when there is no food in the GI tract, the essential problem is that the blood glucose level must be maintained for the survival of the brain and nervous system, which can only use glucose as an energy source. If your blood sugar (glucose) level falls too low you become dizzy and feel faint. Glycogen stores are your first line of defence, and supply your body's glucose needs for several hours when your GI tract is empty – pointing out the importance of carbohydrates in the diet. If fasting continues, protein and to a lesser extent fat are used to produce the glucose needed by the nervous system. Meanwhile, the other organs and tissues of the body go into a glucose-sparing mode and utilize fat as an energy source.

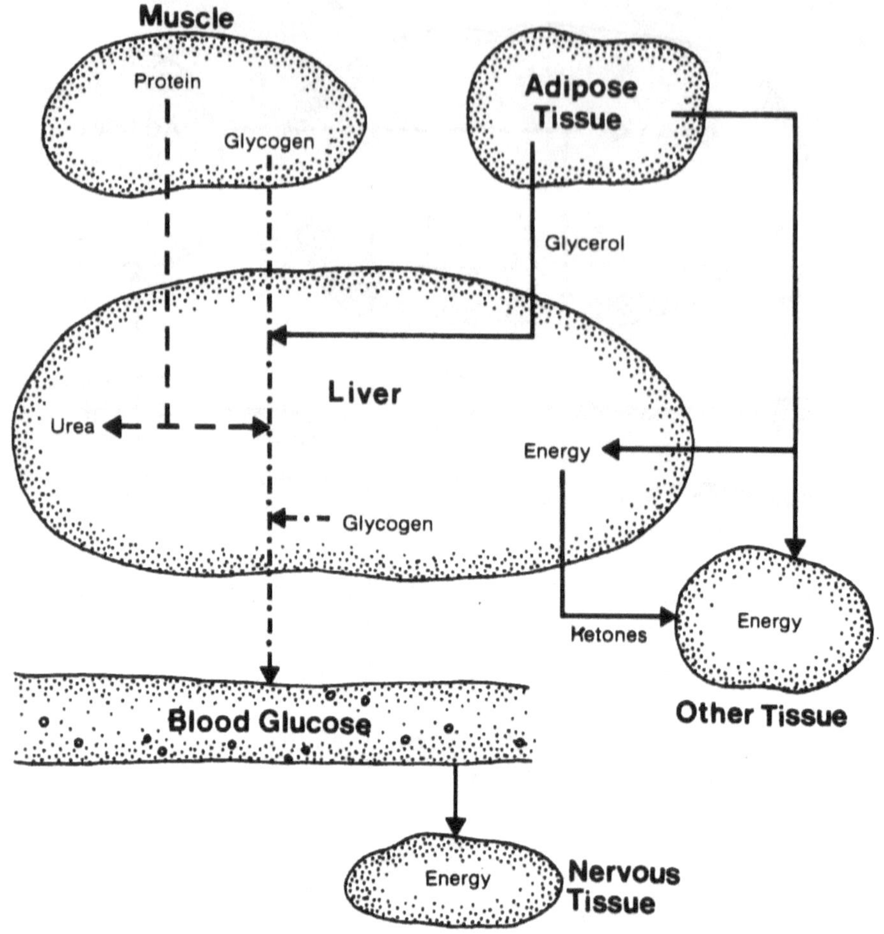

Figure 5.2: Metabolic Pathways - Post-Absorptive Stage

Our Disastrous Eating Habits

Food is far more than just an energy source. Foods are made up of seven basic constituents: carbohydrates, proteins, fats, vitamins, minerals, fibre and water. (Some nutritionists would add phytonutrients to this list – but more on this later.) For healthy bodies we need to eat the correct quantity and proportion of all these components. We need protein, carbohydrates and fats, for growth, repair and energy. We need vitamins and minerals, albeit in relatively small quantities, so they can perform their vital roles in the thousands of biochemical reactions in our body. Fibre, the broad name given to the things we eat that our bodies cannot digest, is needed to assist our digestive system.

Fortunately, in most industrialized countries stores have all the foods we need - and in abundance. Yet most nutritionists agree that a great many people in developed countries are not eating well enough to sustain good health. In many countries diets are too high in fat – with an average of 40 percent of the calories consumed from fat – contributing to atherosclerosis. Another culprit is sugar. In many modern countries approximately 50 kilograms of sugar per year per person is consumed, totalling an unhealthy, nutritionally empty, 500 calories per day. This large intake of sugar lead to obvious ills, such as obesity and tooth decay.

Add to this the increased use of processed and convenience foods, the proliferation of nutritional misinformation and deceptive advertising, and it is clear that most people must improve their understanding of nutrition in order to eat properly.

Nutrients, Micronutrients and Phytonutrients

Before we begin let us define some terms. Nutrients and micronutrients are the components of foods that are essential to human life. Proteins, carbohydrates and fats are nutrients. Some nutritionists refer to proteins, carbohydrates and fats as "macronutrients," and call vitamins and minerals "micronutrients" because they are present in foods in much smaller amounts than macronutrients. More recently, a new grouping of naturally occurring plant-based chemicals, called phytochemicals, or phytonutrients by some nutritionists, have been identified as having many healthful qualities, but unlike traditional macronutrients and micronutrients, phytonutrients are not needed by humans to live; i.e., their absence will not necessarily result in metabolic problems, or a deficiency disease. In the sections that follow we will discuss proteins, carbohydrates, fats, vitamins and minerals, and phytonutrients in some detail.

Proteins are Building Blocks

Proteins are molecules of amino acids that are required for cell maintenance and repair, as well as for the regulation of a wide range of bodily functions. Humans need 22 amino acids in order to live. Our bodies can make 14 of the amino acids on their own, but eight of them, named the essential amino acids, must be acquired from the foods we eat.

Some foods have all the amino acids needed to build other proteins. These are called complete proteins. Nearly every animal food, including dairy products, eggs, meat, poultry and fish are complete proteins because they contain all eight-essential amino acids. Soy is the only plant-based food that has all eight essential-amino acids. Other plant-based protein sources lack one or more essential amino acids (i.e., amino acids that the body can not either create, or manufacture by modifying other amino acids.) These incomplete proteins are found in legumes, grains, nuts, and seeds. However, consuming combinations of foods that have incomplete proteins can provide the same complete protein end effect as animal protein. For a complete-protein meal, simply eat any of the incomplete proteins with another but different incomplete protein, such as eating legumes with grains, or legumes with nuts or seeds, or grains with nuts or seeds. Examples of some healthy plant-protein combinations (that provide complete protein) are pasta and beans, rice and lentils, corn and beans, bean soup with whole-grain bread, split-pea soup with whole-grain bread, peanut butter on whole-grain bread, and tortillas with refried beans.

Around the world, millions of people do not get enough protein. Protein malnutrition can cause growth failure, loss of muscle mass, decreased immunity, weakening of the heart and respiratory system, and in some cases death. Whereas, in developed countries, getting the minimum daily requirement of protein is usually not a problem, because almost any reasonable diet will provide most of us with sufficient protein.

Adults need about 0.79 grams of protein for every kilogram of body weight per day to keep from slowly breaking down their own tissue. (That translates as approximately 0.36 grams of protein per pound of body weight.) A case in point, an adult weighing 11 stone (70 kg) requires about (0.79 x 70), or 55 grams of protein per day. How much protein is in food? Here a few examples: There are approximately seven grams of protein in 30 grams of beef, poultry, fish, cheese or peanuts. Soybeans pack 10 grams of protein per 30 grams. Most other beans and lentils contain about six grams of protein per 30 grams. There are roughly three grams of protein in 30 grams of whole-grain cereal, and milk has one gram of protein per 30 mL.

Understand that foods are rarely straight protein. Some high-protein foods, such as marbled beef and whole milk, also have lots of unhealthy saturated fat. Therefore, when you eat meat, eat the leanest cuts, and when you consume dairy products, choose skim or low-fat versions. On the other hand, beans, nuts, and whole grains offer high-quality (albeit incomplete) protein with little saturated fat - but with lots of healthful fibre and micronutrients.

You Need Carbohydrates

Carbohydrates provide your body with its basic fuel, the energy your cells need to survive. The staple of most diets around the world, carbohydrates provide essential vitamins and minerals, fibre, and numerous beneficial compounds (phytonutrients) that promote good health.

The simplest carbohydrate is glucose. Glucose, also called "blood sugar" and "dextrose," flows in the bloodstream so that it is available to every cell in your body. Your body's cells absorb glucose and convert it into energy to drive the cell. Glucose is a simple sugar, meaning that it tastes sweet. Some other simple sugars are sucrose, also known as "white sugar," fructose, the main sugar in fruits, and lactose, the sugar found in milk. They all taste sweet, and most are digested and enter your bloodstream quickly. When you eat fruit or drink milk, however, the natural sugar comes with vitamins, minerals (and fibre in the case of fruit); whereas the simple sugars in candy, for example, are nothing but nutritionally-empty calories.

Then there are the more complex carbohydrates. Most grains (wheat, corn, oats, rice) and foods like potatoes, pasta and plantains are complex carbohydrates. In general, but not always, complex carbohydrates are digested more slowly than simple carbohydrates, and take much longer to enter your bloodstream. Most of us have heard that eating complex carbohydrates is good, and eating sugar-loaded foods is a bad. The reason is that simple sugars require little digestion, and when you eat a sweet food, such as a candy, your blood glucose level rises rapidly. In response, your pancreas secretes a large amount of insulin to keep your blood glucose levels from rising too high. The large insulin response in turn tends to cause your blood sugar to fall to levels that are too low. As a consequence, about three to five hours after consuming sweets you feel lethargic and hungry. Many people react to this by eating yet another sweet, which can start a series of glucose and then insulin surges. None of this is experienced after eating most complex carbohydrates, or a balanced meal, because the digestion and absorption processes are much slower. series

Glycemic Index

Thinking of carbohydrates as complex or simple, as good or bad, is outdated. More recently, a system has been devised to classify carbohydrates. The system, called the glycemic index (GI), measures the effect a carbohydrate has on your blood sugar – quantifying how rapidly and to what level your blood sugar rises after you eat a food containing carbohydrates, compared to a reference food (usually glucose or white bread). For instance, a candy bar, which is digested rapidly has a high GI and causes an almost immediate jump in your blood sugar; whereas, lentil soup is digested more slowly and has a low GI. The factors that influence a food's GI are:

a) <u>Fibre</u> prevents the rapid digestion of the carbohydrates in food and slows the discharge of sugar molecules into the blood stream. Higher fibre content results in a lower GI.

b) <u>Coarsely-ground grains</u> are digested more slowly and, therefore, have lower GI values than finely-ground grains.

c) <u>Less-processed</u> carbohydrates, such whole-grain foods where the fibre, bran and germ are intact, are digested more slowly than highly-processed carbohydrates. It follows, therefore, that less processing usually results in a lower GI.

d) <u>Unripe</u> fruits and vegetables contain less sugar and have a lower GI than ripe varieties.

e) The <u>more acid or fat</u> a food has, the slower its carbohydrates are digested and absorbed into the blood stream. More acid and fat in a food mean a lower GI.

These factors sometimes lead to unexpected results. For instance, some foods containing simple carbohydrates such as fruit have a lower GI than a complex carbohydrate like the potato.

The glycemic index uses a scale of 0 to 100, with foods that cause the most rapid rise in blood sugar having the highest values. In this book and many others, glucose is the arbitrary reference food, and is assigned a GI = 100. (For a given food, a GI less than 56 is considered low, a GI = 56 to 69 is medium, and a GI greater than 69 is high.) Note that foods that contain little or no carbohydrate (such as meat, fish, eggs, avocado, wine, beer and other alcoholic beverages) do not have GI values.

Glycemic Load

Some food scientists have come to recognize that a food's GI value alone does not provide enough information to judge how a particular food will affect your blood sugar. This is because the GI does not take into account how much carbohydrate is in a food serving, and your blood sugar level is influenced by both the quality of the carbohydrate (GI) and the quantity of carbohydrate you eat. With this in mind, researchers developed a new guideline called the glycemic load (GL) which takes into account both a food's GI and the quantity of carbohydrate the food contains. A food's GL is calculated by multiplying the food's GI by the number of carbohydrate grams in a serving. For a given food, a GL less 11 is considered low, a GL = 11 to 19 medium, and a GL greater than 19 is high. Most people consume 60 to 180 GL units per day, with a GL of about 100 for a typical diet.

Table 5.1 (on the next page) presents GI and GL values for some common foods. Most of the data are from the on-line database of the University of Sidney (Australia). The difference between a food's GI and GL is illustrated by a simple example. Table 5.1 indicates watermelon has a GI = 72, quite high. In this case, however, GI alone is misleading because watermelon only has about six grams of carbohydrate per serving. (Watermelon is almost entirely water, with some fibre and a small quantity of carbohydrate.) So a typical serving of watermelon, has a GL = GI x (net carb grams) = 0.72 x 6 = 4.3, which is quite low. (Note in the calculation, watermelon's GI value has been converted from 72% to the decimal equivalent 0.72.)

Some diet book authors claim a food's GI and in some cases GL are the most important guidelines to use when planning a weight-loss diet. But consider the following: Pears (not shown in Table 5.1) are forbidden by some diets because of a relatively high GI = 40. However, a medium size pear weighing about four ounces has a GL = 4, quite low. Now consider a four ounce serving of peanuts with a much lower GI = 14, and an even lower GL = 2. For people on a reducing diet, based only on Glycemic Index or Load, a snack of peanuts appears to be a better choice than a pear. A medium-size pear, however, contains only 70 kcalories, while four ounces of peanuts are loaded with about 650 kcalories! Pears and peanuts are both healthy foods, but the extra 580 kcalories in peanuts are certainly not going to help you lose weight.

The focus on a food's GI can lead to limiting healthful foods that may have a high GI by themselves, but when eaten in combination with other foods are not a problem. A nutritious baked potato may have a high GI, but when eaten as part of a complete meal is digested more slowly than its GI value would indicate. The main point is that if you use GI or GL values as the sole factor when selecting your food, you could be eliminating very healthy foods, and eating too many calories and often too much fat as well. It is important, therefore, to appreciate that a food's GI and GL numbers only allow you to evaluate how a food's carbohydrate content affects your blood sugar level. Because your body performs better when your blood sugar remains relatively constant, we should be aware of a food's GL rank and consider it when planning your eating pattern. But there are other important factors that must also be taken into account, such as getting the micronutrients we need from a variety of foods, including carbohydrates, and staying within your caloric allowance.

Food	Glycemic Index (%)	Serving Size	Net Carbs	Glycemic Load
Strawberries	40	150 g	3	1
Peanuts	14	100 g	9	1
Peach	42	1 large (120 g)	8	3
Carrot	92	1 large (80 g)	4	4
Lentils	28	150 g	15	4
Orange	48	1 medium (120 g)	9	4
Watermelon	72	120 g	6	4
Apple	40	1 medium (138 g)	15	6
Ice Cream	65	1 scoop (50 g)	10	7
Bread (whole wheat)	73	1 slice (30 g)	11	8
Grapes	46	120 g	18	8
Bread (white)	70	1 slice (30 g)	13	9
Corn (sweet)	59	1 ear (80 g)	16	9
Banana	50	1 large (120 g)	24	12
Oatmeal	58	225 g	21	12
Sweet potato	50	1 medium (150 g)	26	13
Spaghetti	45	180 g	44	20
Potato (baked)	94	1 medium (150 g)	22	21
Rice (brown)	50	130 g	48	24
Raisins	64	1 sm box (60 g)	43	28
Rice (white)	72	130 g	42	30
Candy bar	55	1 bar (113 g)	64	35
Glucose	100	50 g	50	50

Table 5.1: Glycemic Rank of Common Foods

In summary, **carbohydrates are neither all good nor all bad.** Remember good carbohydrates provide needed micronutrients. You should try to get the bulk of your calories from the good carbohydrates, i.e., from fruits, from vegetables and from whole grains such as whole-grain cereal, whole-wheat bread, whole-grain pasta, whole-old-fashioned oats, brown rice, bulgur, millet, and hulled barley.

Cholesterol and Triglyceride

Atherosclerosis has been linked to both blood cholesterol and triglyceride levels. Both fatty substances are found in the plaque on the walls of clogged arteries. There are two types of cholesterol: high-density cholesterol (HDL), the "good" cholesterol, and low-density cholesterol (LDL), the "bad" cholesterol. You should have your cholesterol and triglyceride levels measured during a regular medical check-up and should know and understand the readings. At this writing, the desirable readings for otherwise healthy individuals are as follows:

- **Total cholesterol level should be less than 200 mg/dl.**

- **High-density cholesterol (HDL) should be greater than 40 mg/dl.**

- **Low-density cholesterol (LDL) should be less than 130 mg/dl.**

- **Triglyceride reading should be less than 150 mg/dl.**

For people who have coronary-artery disease, most cardiologists insist that the total cholesterol level be less than 160 mg/dl and the even more important LDL cholesterol be less than 100 mg/dl. Recently, cardiologists have been urging patients with coronary-artery disease to reduce their LDL even further to below 70 mg/dl.

Often, cholesterol and triglyceride levels can be reduced by adhering to the eating recommendations summarized at the end of the section that immediately follows, called "Fats in Foods." Where a low-fat diet alone does not work, people with high cholesterol and or high triglyceride levels, may be prescribed cholesterol-lowering medication by their physician. For more information on this important subject, visit the American Heart Association website:.

Fats Found in Foods

Fats are found in vegetable oil, seeds and nuts, meat and fish, and dairy products, as well as in foods like potato chips and french fries (that are cooked in oil), cookies, cake, and so on. There are certain fats you absolutely need to survive (the essential-fatty acids), and others you would do well to drastically limit (saturated fats) or avoid altogether (trans fats). Chemically, all fatty acids contain carbon chains with hydrogen atoms bonded to the carbon, and all fats have the highest calorie density – containing nine calories per gram (see page 105).

Until recently, the best wisdom was to eat a low-fat, low-cholesterol diet. This advice is now largely out of date. The latest research seems to show that the total amount of fat in the diet may not be linked with disease. **What really matters is the type of fat in your diet.**

Saturated Fats: When all carbon bonds of a fat molecule are filled with hydrogen, a fat is said to be saturated, i.e., saturated with hydrogen atoms. Most saturated fats are animal in origin and are solid at room temperature (good examples are butter and the fat in meats). Generally speaking, you should avoid or at least severely limit your intake of saturated fats because they can raise both your total and bad LDL blood cholesterol levels which increases your chances of getting heart disease.

When hydrogen atoms are missing along the carbon chain the fatty acids are called monounsaturated or polyunsaturated depending on their exact chemical structure.

Monounsaturated fats (also called omega-9 fatty acids) are liquid at room temperature and are known as oils. They are "good fats" and are derived from plant sources, such as vegetable oils, nuts, and seeds. In studies in which monounsaturated fats were eaten in place of carbohydrates, LDL blood cholesterol levels decreased and HDL cholesterol levels increased. Monounsaturated fats are found in high concentrations in canola, olive and peanut oils.

Polyunsaturated fats are also liquid oils at room temperature and in your refrigerator. They are "good fats" and are derived from plant sources, such as vegetable oils, nuts, and seeds. Again, research has demonstrated that when polyunsaturated fats were eaten in place of carbohydrates, LDL blood cholesterol levels decreased and HDL cholesterol levels increased. Polyunsaturated fats are found in high concentrations in sunflower, soybean and corn oils.

Essential-Fatty Acids are class of polyunsaturated fatty acids that our body cannot create. These fats must be obtained from the food you eat. Essential-fatty acids promote absorption of the fat-soluble vitamins A, D, E, and K and are also thought to provide many disease-fighting benefits. Because essential-fatty acids are needed and our body cannot manufacture them, they must come from the food we eat. Essential-fatty acids fall into two groups: omega-3 and omega-6.

Omega-3 fatty acids are relatively hard to find. Foods high in omega-3 fatty acids are walnuts, tofu, flax seeds and oily fish (salmon, mackerel, sardines, trout and albacore tuna). Omega-3 fats are thought to be heart-protective. (In many European countries, but not in the United States, people who have suffered a heart attack and those with coronary-heart disease are often prescribed a fish-oil supplement.)

Omega-6 fatty acids, on the other hand, are more common, easier to find, and are in most oils including sunflower, soybean and corn oils.

Current thinking is that the consumption of omega-6 and omega-3 fatty acids should be in the ratio of 3:1, with about three omega-6 for one omega-3. Many Western diets, however, contain about 15:1, omega-6 to omega-3, which is not good for your health. Although you need omega-6, people generally eat too much of it and not enough omega-3 fat. The American Heart Association recommends that you eat fish (particularly fatty fish) two times a week, as a way to get a more appropriate quantity of omega-3 fatty acids in your diet.

Trans fats are produced when liquid oil is processed into a solid fat. The manufacturing process is called hydrogenation, or partial hydrogenation, and trans fats are an unnatural by-product. Partially-hydrogenated vegetable oils are considered especially unhealthy, because of the resulting trans fatty acids and the added hydrogen saturation. Research indicates that trans fats are even worse than saturated fats because they not only raise bad LDL cholesterol but also lower good HDL cholesterol. Eliminating foods containing partially-hydrogenated oils from your diet is vital to good health.

In summary, it is becoming increasingly clear that saturated and trans fats, increase the risk for certain diseases while monounsaturated and polyunsaturated fats, lower the risk. The key is not to eliminate fat from your diet but to substitute good fats for bad fats, and at the same time try to reduce the total amount of fat consumed because all fats are very high in calories.

Fat Type	Where found
Saturated	Meat, poultry (especially the skin), dairy products, lard, coconut oil, palm oil, cocoa butter
Trans Fats	Fried foods, margarine, snack foods, commercially-baked cake and cookies, and fast foods
Cholesterol	Egg yokes, dairy products, organ meats, fatty and prime meats, poultry skin, shellfish (particularly shrimp)
Polyunsaturated (Omega-3)	Mackerel, salmon, sardines, tuna, canola oil, walnuts, flaxseed, wheat germ
Polyunsaturated (Omega-6)	Corn oil, cottonseed oil, safflower oil, sunflower oil, soybean oil
Monounsaturated (Omega-9)	Canola oil, olive oil, safflower oil (hybrid), sunflower oil (hybrid)

Table 5.2: Fats in Foods

Current scientific thinking regarding fat consumption is as follows:

- **Try to limit the total fat you eat** to no more than 30 percent of your caloric intake.

- **Do not consume foods containing partially-hydrogenated vegetable oil** because they are high in trans fats. This includes commercially prepared baked goods, snack foods, and processed foods, including fast foods. To be safe, assume these products contain trans fats unless otherwise labelled.

- **Limit saturated fats**, i.e., any fat of animal origin, to 10 percent of your caloric intake. Have meat less often, and when serving meat use lean cuts and trim the fat. Eat fish and poultry (white meat, without the skin) more frequently. Use skim (fat-free) milk and fat-free dairy products in place of whole milk. (Coconut and palm oil should also be avoided because they are saturated fats.)

- When consuming fat, **choose foods containing monounsaturated fats** like olive oil and canola oil, **and foods rich in polyunsaturated omega-6 and omega-3 fatty acids.**

- Try to balance your intake essential fatty acids by eating more omega-3 fatty acids, found in walnuts, tofu, certain seeds and oily fish such as salmon, sardines and tuna.

Vitamins and Minerals

The following is a listing of vitamins and minerals complete with a brief discussion of their function in your body, what foods supply the particular micronutrient, and the Recommended Dietary Allowance (RDA) - which is a reference number developed by the United States Food and Drug Administration to help consumers determine how much of a specific micronutrient a food contains. Summaries of the RDAs for vitamins and minerals are shown in Table 5.3 (on page 90) and Table 5.4 (on page 94). that RDAs are frequently gender and age dependent, and pregnant and nursing women most often have special micronutrient needs.

Because of the rapid expansion of scientific knowledge regarding the role of micronutrients in human health, the U.S. Food and Drug Administration, in partnership with Health Canada, periodically assesses and updates the recommended Daily Values. The following contains the recommended RDAs as of April 2006 for the vitamins and minerals discussed.

Vitamin A is a collection of fat-soluble compounds that play an important role in vision, bone growth, reproduction, cell division, and help prevent or fight off infections. Vitamin A also promotes healthy surface linings of the eyes, respiratory, urinary, and intestinal tracts, and also helps maintain the integrity of skin and mucous membranes. Using the long-established International Unit (IU) measure for the recommended dietary allowance (RDA), adult men and women need 3,000 and 2,330 IU (as retinol) per day respectively. However, the new RDA measure for vitamin A is the microgram (mcg), which translates for men and women as 900 and 700 mcg per day. Foods rich in vitamin A are orange-coloured vegetables such as carrots, sweet potatoes and pumpkin; dark-green-leafy vegetables like spinach, collards and romaine lettuce; and orange-coloured fruits such as mango, cantaloupe and apricots; and red peppers and tomatoes. One medium-size carrot supplies approximately 270 percent of your RDA.

Vitamin D is a fat-soluble vitamin. Briefly, vitamin D is important in assisting the absorption of calcium, in forming strong bones and teeth and preventing deficiency diseases such as rickets and osteomalacia. For most adults, an adequate intake of vitamin D is 200 to 600 IU (which is equivalent to 5 to 15 mcg per day). In addition, your body can make vitamin D after exposure to sunshine. Good food sources include salt-water fish such as herring, salmon, sardines and fish-liver oils, as well as fortified milk and cereals. Small quantities are also found in egg yokes, veal and beef. 250 mL of fortified milk supplies about 25 percent of your daily needs.

Vitamin	Age					
	19-30	31-50	51-70	70+	Preg	Lact
A (mcg)	700	700	700	700	770	1300
D (mcg)	5	5	10	15	5	5
E (mcg)	15	15	15	15	15	19
K (mcg)	90	90	90	90	90	90
C (mg)	75	75	75	75	85	120
B_1 (mg)	1.1	1.1	1.1	1.1	1.4	1.4
B_2 (mg)	1.1	1.1	1.1	1.1	1.4	1.6
B_3 (mg)	14	14	14	14	18	17
B_5 (mg)	5	5	5	5	6	7
B_6 (mg)	1.3	1.3	1.5	1.5	1.9	2.0
B_7 (mcg)	30	30	30	30	30	35
B_9 (mcg)	400	400	400	400	600	500
B_{12} (mcg)	2.4	2.4	2.4	2.4	2.6	2.8

Table 5.3: Vitamin RDA for Women

Values for vitamins D, K, B_5 and B_7 are Adequate Intake. Preg = pregnant Lact = lactating mcg = micrograms per day mg = milligrams per day.

Vitamin E is a fat-soluble vitamin that is a powerful antioxidant and acts to protect cells against the effects of free radicals, which are potentially damaging by-products of energy metabolism. Research is underway to determine if vitamin E, through its ability to limit the production of free radicals, might help prevent or delay the development of cardiovascular disease and some cancers. For adults, the RDA for vitamin E is 22.5 IU (as d-alpha-tocopherol) which is equal to 15 mcg per day. Foods rich in vitamin E are vegetable oils, nuts, seeds, milk fat, egg yolks, liver, dark-green-leafy vegetables, and whole-grain foods. Approximately 12 almonds provide 100 percent of your RDA for vitamin E.

Vitamin K is another fat-soluble vitamin, and is known as the clotting vitamin, because without it blood would not clot. Some studies also indicate that it helps maintain strong bones in the elderly. Adequate intake of vitamin K for men is 120 mcg per day and for women 90 mcg per day. Good sources are dark-green-leafy vegetables, soybean, cottonseed, canola, and olive oil. People who eat these foods as part of a balanced diet should easily get enough vitamin K.

Vitamin C is a water-soluble, antioxidant vitamin. It is important in forming collagen, a protein that gives structure to bones, cartilage, muscle, and blood vessels. Vitamin C also aids in the absorption of iron, and helps maintain capillaries, bones, and teeth. The RDA for vitamin C is 90 milligrams (mg) per day for men and 75 mg per day for women. Foods rich in vitamin C are citrus fruits and juices, kiwifruit, strawberries, cantaloupe, broccoli, peppers, tomatoes, cabbage potatoes, and dark-green-leafy vegetables. 180 mL of orange juice supplies 100 percent of a man's RDA.

Vitamin B is actually a complex of different water-soluble vitamins that often exist in the same foods. They perform an important role in our metabolism, in maintaining muscle tone along our digestive tract and in the health of our nervous system, skin, hair, eyes, mouth, and liver. The B complex vitamins are: vitamin B_1 (thiamine), vitamin B_2 (riboflavin), vitamin B_3 (niacin), vitamin B_5 (pantothenic acid), vitamin B_6 (pyridoxine), vitamin B_7 (biotin), vitamin B_9 (folic acid), and vitamin B_{12} (cyanocobalamin). Many cereals are fortified with all the B vitamins. Depending on the brand, one serving of a fortified cereal provides from 25 to 100 percent of the RDA for all the B vitamins (except vitamin B_7 biotin).

Vitamin B_1 (thiamine) plays a vital role in the proper operation of your nervous system. Your body also needs B_1 to convert carbohydrates into sugar and then energy. The RDA for men is 1.2 mg per day and 1.1 mg per day for women. Vitamin B_1 is found in meat, wheat germ, whole-grains cereals and breads, in enriched cereals and breads, in beans, nuts and seeds, and in dark-green-leafy vegetables.

Vitamin B_2 (riboflavin) also has a crucial role in certain metabolic reactions, particularly the conversion of carbohydrates into energy. Riboflavin is also an important antioxidant. The RDA is 1.3 mg per day for men and 1.1 mg per day for women. The best sources of riboflavin are brewer's yeast, almonds, organ meats, whole grains, wheat germ, wild rice, mushrooms, soybeans, milk, yogurt, eggs, broccoli, and spinach. In addition, flours and cereals are often fortified with riboflavin.

Vitamin B_3 (niacin) helps clear toxic and harmful chemicals from your body. It also assists in the production of various hormones. Niacin improves your circulation and reduces blood cholesterol levels. The RDA is 16 mg per day for men and 14 mg per day for women. Foods containing significant amounts of niacin are liver, meat, poultry, fish, whole-grains and nuts.

Vitamin B₅ (pantothenic acid) is necessary for a variety of life-sustaining tasks such as generating energy from food, synthesizing essential fats, and the function of your adrenal glands. Adequate intake of vitamin B_5 for adults is 5 mg per day. Good sources include organ meats, eggs, fish and shellfish, poultry, soybeans, beans, dairy foods, avocado, and mushrooms.

Vitamin B₆ (pyridoxine) is needed for protein and red-blood cell metabolism. Your body also requires vitamin B_6 to make haemoglobin. For men and women up to 50 years old, the RDA is 1.3 mg per day. After 50, the RDA increases to 1.7 mg per day for men and 1.5 mg for women. Vitamin B_6 is found in a wide variety of foods including fortified cereals, beans, meat, poultry, fish, and some fruits and vegetables.

Vitamin B₇ (biotin) functions as a coenzyme in the synthesis of fat, glycogen and amino acids. An adequate intake of biotin is 30 mcg per day. A varied diet should provide enough biotin for most people. Liver, yeast and egg yokes are particularly rich food sources. It is also found in smaller amounts in fruit, meat and cheese.

Vitamin B₉ (folate or folic acid) helps produce and maintain new cells which is particularly important during periods of rapid cell division and growth such as in infancy and during pregnancy. Folate is needed to make DNA and RNA, the building blocks of cells. It is also thought to prevent DNA changes that may lead to cancer. For most adults, the RDA of folate is 400 mcg per day. Of course, woman who are expecting or nursing need more folate.   Cooked dry beans and peas, peanuts, oranges, dark-green-leafy vegetables and green peas are folate-rich foods.

Vitamin B₁₂ (cyanocobalamin) enables your body to manufacture healthy red-blood cells. It also assists in the transmission of electrical signals between nerve cells. The recommended dietary allowance is 2.4 mcg per day. Vitamin B_{12} is found in fortified cereals, meat, fish and poultry.

Calcium is a mineral with several important functions. Most of the calcium in your body is used to support the structure of your bones and teeth. A small amount of calcium is in your blood, muscle, and the fluid between your cells. Calcium is also needed for muscle contraction, blood vessel contraction and expansion, the secretion of hormones and enzymes, and sending messages through the nervous system. For most adults, adequate intake is 1000 mg per day. Foods rich in calcium are milk, yogurt, natural cheeses (such as cheddar, Swiss and mozzarella), canned fish with soft bones such as salmon and sardines, and dark-green-leafy vegetables. 250 mL of fat-free milk contains about 30 percent of your RDA.

Chromium is important in the metabolism of fats and carbohydrates and in controlling blood sugar levels. It is an activator of several enzymes needed to drive numerous chemical reactions necessary to life. For men and women up to 50 years old, an adequate intake of chromium is 35 and 25 mcg per day respectively. After 50, the recommended adequate intake drops to 30 mcg per day for men and 20 for women. Whole grains, ready-to-eat bran cereals, seafood, green beans, broccoli, prunes, nuts, peanut butter, and potatoes are rich in chromium. 120 mL container of chopped broccoli provides about 35 percent of your chromium RDA.

Iodine is a basic component of the thyroid hormone that regulates your metabolic rate. Lack of iodine can cause a number of physical and mental abnormalities. RDA for adult men and women is 150 mcg per day. Iodized salt, sea food and plants grown in iodine-rich soil are good sources of iodine. 100 grams of cooked haddock contains about 140 mcg of iodine.

Iron is an important mineral that aids the transport of oxygen in your body and is also needed for the regulation of cell growth. An iron deficiency limits oxygen delivery to cells, resulting in fatigue and decreased immunity. The RDA for iron is 8 mg per day for men and 18 mg per day for pre-menopausal women. Foods rich in iron are shrimp, clams, mussels, oysters, sardines, lean meats (especially beef), organ meats, turkey (dark meat), spinach, cooked dry beans, peas, lentils, and whole-grain breads and cereals. 100 grams of beef liver has approximately 55 percent of your iron RDA, and fortified cereals can provide from 50 to 100 percent of your RDA.

Magnesium is needed for hundreds of biochemical reactions in your body. It helps maintain normal muscle and nerve function, keeps heart rhythm steady, supports a healthy immune system, and keeps bones strong. The RDA is 420 mg per day for men and 320 for women. Dark-green-leafy vegetables, fish, some beans and peas, nuts and seeds, and whole grains are good sources of magnesium. 120 mL container of cooked spinach has 75 mg of magnesium.

Phosphorus in combination with calcium is necessary for the formation of bones and teeth. Phosphorus is also involved in the metabolism of fats, carbohydrates and proteins, and in the effective utilization of many of the B vitamins. The RDA for adults is 700 mg per day. Rich sources of phosphorus are dairy products, meat, and fish. Phosphorus is also present in most soft drinks. Generally, a diet that provides adequate amounts of calcium and protein also provides a sufficient amount of phosphorus.

Mineral	Age					
	19 to 30	31 to 50	51 to70	70+	Preg	Lact
Calcium (mg)	1000	1000	1200	1200	1000	1000
Chromium (mcg)	25	25	20	20	30	45
Copper (mcg)	900	900	900	900	1000	1300
Fluoride (mg)	3	3	3	3	3	3
Iodine (mcg)	150	150	150	150	220	290
Iron (mg)	18	18	8	8	27	9
Magnesium (mg)	310	320	320	320	355	315
Manganese (mg)	1.8	1.8	1.8	1.8	2.0	2.6
Molybdenum (mcg)	45	45	45	45	50	50
Phosphorus (mg)	700	700	700	700	700	700
Potassium (mg)	4700	4700	4700	4700	4700	5100
Selenium (mcg)	55	55	55	55	60	70
Zinc (mg)	8	8	8	8	8	8

Table 5.4: Recommended Dietary Allowances (RDA) for Minerals

Preg = pregnant   Lact = lactating mcg = micrograms per day mg = milligrams per day. Calcium, chromium, fluoride & manganese values are Adequate Intake.

Potassium is involved in proper nerve function, muscle control and blood pressure regulation. (People engaged in vigorous exercise may need more potassium to replace that lost during exercise.) Low potassium levels can cause muscle cramping and cardiovascular irregularities. Adequate intake for men and women is 4700 mg per day. Potassium-rich foods include baked white or sweet potatoes, cooked leafy greens, winter (orange) squash, bananas, oranges, dried fruits (such as apricots and prunes), and cooked dry beans and lentils. A medium-size baked potato contains about 600 mg of potassium.

Selenium is an essential trace element that assists enzymes involved in antioxidant protection and thyroid hormone metabolism. The RDA is 55 mcg per day for men and women. The most important sources in American diets are meats, fish and grains. 100 grams of cooked cod fish provides about 36 mcg of selenium.

Zinc is an essential mineral that stimulates the activity of approximately 100 enzymes that promote biochemical reactions in your body. Zinc supports a healthy immune system needed for wound healing, and helps maintain your sense of taste and smell. The RDA for zinc is 11 mg per day for men and 8 mg per day for women. Oysters contain more zinc per serving than any other food. Other good sources are red meat, poultry, beans, nuts, certain seafood, whole grains, dairy products and fortified breakfast cereals which can provide from 50 to 100 percent of your RDA.

Phytonutrients Emerge

Phytonutrients are not vitamins or minerals. Rather they are the beneficial compounds that give fruits and vegetables their many colours. "Phyto" comes from the Greek word for "plant," and that is where phytonutrients are found - in plant foods such as fruits, vegetables, whole grains, dried beans, nuts and seeds. Unlike traditional macronutrients and micronutrients (protein, fat, vitamins and minerals), phytonutrients are not necessary for life; i.e., they are not required for normal metabolism and their absence will not result in a deficiency disease. Despite this, research is expanding as evidence grows that phytonutrients have many beneficial qualities such as assisting the function of the immune system, reducing inflammation, acting directly against viruses, and playing a crucial role in preventing or reducing the risk of a number of chronic ailments, including heart disease, diabetes and cancer.

One of the most important roles of phytonutrients is as an antioxidant. Free radicals, which are by-products of energy metabolism, can damage cells and are thought to contribute to the development of cardiovascular disease and cancer. When antioxidant molecules encounter free radicals they neutralize them - limiting the damage. Your body needs more antioxidants as you grow older, because your body's ability to repair itself diminishes as you age. Antioxidants can also help to prevent cell damage by environmental carcinogens.

Scientists understanding of phytonutrients is still in its infancy. Despite this, about one thousand phytonutrients have been identified to date and with ever expanding research new compounds are continually being discovered and organized into classes. The best known phytonutrient classes are carotenoids and polyphenols.

Carotenoids are contained in the yellow, orange, and red pigment in fruits and vegetables, as well as in dark-green-leafy vegetables (where the usual yellow colour is masked by the vegetable's green pigment).

Some of the phytonutrients within the carotenoids class are alpha-carotene (contained in carrots); beta-carotene (in broccoli, sweet potato, pumpkin and carrots); beta-cryptoxanthin (in citrus fruits, peaches and apricots); lutein (in leafy greens such as kale, spinach and turnip greens); lycopene (in tomatoes, tomato paste, guava, pink grapefruit and watermelon); and zeaxanthin (in green vegetables, eggs and citrus fruit).

Polyphenol compounds are natural components of a wide variety of plants. Foods rich in polyphenols include apples, red wine, red grapes, grape juice, strawberries, raspberries, blueberries, cranberries, onions, tea, and certain nuts. Polyphenols are further subdivided into flavonoids and nonflavonoids.

Some phytonutrients in the flavonoids subgroup are anthocyanins (in fruits); catechins (found in tea and red wine); flavanones (in citrus fruit) flavones (in most fruits and vegetables); flavonols (in most fruits, vegetables, tea and red wine); and isoflavones (in soybeans). The nonflavonoids subgroup contains ellagic acid (contained in strawberries, bilberries and raspberries).

Guidelines for Healthy Eating

No single food can supply all the nutrients you need in the amounts you need. The most important factors in nutrition are variety, variety, variety! **Variety is the key to a nutritious diet**. As a means of setting strategies for food selection for the general population, many nations have issued dietary food guides similar to the U.S. Department of Health and Human Services Dietary 2005 Guidelines (e.g., Health Canada) that describe a healthy diet as one that:

- Emphasizes fruits, vegetables, whole grains, and fat-free or low-fat milk products.

- Includes fish, poultry, lean meats, beans and nuts.

- Is low in saturated fats, trans fats, cholesterol, salt (sodium) and added sugars.

The guidelines encourage adults to consume a variety of nutrient-dense foods and beverages within their caloric needs. In 2005 the afore mentioned U.S.

government agency recommended how much should be eaten from each of the basic food groups, subgroups and oils (i.e., from fruits, vegetables, grains, meat and beans, milk, and oils) to meet your caloric goal – whether you are trying to lose weight or maintain weight. This information is displayed, using the metric system of units, in Table 5.5. The table also shows the elective calorie allowance available within each calorie level. Elective calories are those remaining after we account for the calories consumed eating the recommended amount of food from all the food groups. (Note, in the daily calorie goal column, you should use either your weight loss or weight maintenance calorie level, as explained later in Chapter 6, "Weight Control.")

The Basic Food Groups

In this section we describe the various food groups, indicate what constitutes a serving size, and focus on the best foods within each group. The foods in **bold font** are generally the most nutrient-dense foods – the best of the best.

Fruit Group: Includes fresh, frozen, canned and dried fruits and fruit juices. Usually, <u>one serving</u> consists of approximately 130 grams of fresh, frozen or canned fruit, or 75 grams of dried fruit, or 250 mL of 100 percent fruit juice. This group can be divided further into citrus fruits, berries and grapes, and other fruits.

    Citrus fruits: There are many excellent citrus choices including **oranges, grapefruit, lemons, limes, kiwifruit and kumquats**. All are low calorie foods that contain a negligible amount of fat and cholesterol, are high in vitamin C, and most have significant amounts of vitamin A, potassium and dietary fibre.

    Berries & grapes: Among the fruits in this grouping are **blackberries, bilberries, raspberries, strawberries, cranberries, gooseberries, purple grapes, black currents, raisins, and cherries**. Every fresh berry and grape is low calorie, with no fat or cholesterol, and all have small amounts of multiple micronutrients and a fair amount of dietary fibre. (Strawberries are also rich in vitamin C.) Some researchers claim that the blue and black-coloured berries are packed with more disease-fighting antioxidants than any other fruit or vegetable. Of course, the dark-red and purple grapes contain the phytonutrient flavonols, the same antioxidant believed to give red wine its heart-protecting benefits.

    Other fruits: This large subgroup includes a number of healthy foods such as **apples, apricots, bananas, cantaloupe, figs, mangos, papayas,**

peaches, pears, pineapples, plums, prunes and watermelon. Again, all are low calorie, contain no fat or cholesterol, and are loaded with vitamins, minerals and phytonutrients. In addition, apples, apricots, figs, peaches, pears, pineapples, plums, prunes are good sources of dietary fibre. Cantaloupe is also high in vitamin C and watermelon contains the phytonutrient lycopene.

Daily kcal Goal	Fruits Serving	Vegetable Servings	Grains Serving	Meat, Fish, etc	Milk Serving	Oils (mL)	Approx Elective kcalories
1000	1	1	3	2	2	15	170
1200	1	1.5	4	3	2	20	170
1400	1.5	1.5	5	4	2	20	170
1600	1.5	2	5	5	3	25	130
1800	1.5	2.5	6	5	3	25	200
2000	2	2.5	6	5.5	3	30	270
2200	2	3	7	6	3	30	290
2400	2	3	8	6.5	3	35	360
2600	2	3.5	9	6.5	3	39	410
2800	2.5	3.5	10	7	3	39	430
3000	2.5	4	10	7	3	49	510
3200	2.5	4	10	7	3	54	650

Table 5.5: Recommended Servings/Portion Sizes for Different Food Groups

Vegetable Group: Includes fresh, frozen, dried and canned vegetables and vegetable juices. In general, _one serving_ from the vegetable group consists of about 130 grams of raw or cooked vegetables, or 250 mL of vegetable juice. This group can be broken down further into dark-green-leafy vegetables, orange-coloured vegetables, starchy vegetables and other vegetables.

Dark-green-leafy vegetables: Every food in this category (which includes **bok choy, collard greens, kale, mustard greens, romaine**

lettuce, spinach, Swiss chard and turnip greens) is low calorie with no fat or cholesterol, and is packed with micronutrients, especially vitamins A and C, calcium, iron, potassium and folate, as well as dietary fibre.

Orange-coloured vegetables: The best in this subgroup are **carrots, orange-bell peppers, pumpkin, sweet potatoes, yams and winter squash**. All have negligible fat and cholesterol and are high in vitamin A, potassium and dietary fibre.

Starchy vegetables: This grouping overlaps somewhat with the orange-coloured vegetable subgroup and the grains group. Among the foods included are **white potatoes, sweet potatoes, yams, yellow corn, and brown rice**. These vegetables are generally high in complex carbohydrates, B vitamins, potassium and dietary fibre.

Other vegetables: This extensive category contains **asparagus, broccoli, brussels sprouts, cabbage, cauliflower, celery, cucumber, fennel, green beans, parsley, and summer squash**. The preceding are low calorie foods that contain a negligible amount of fat and cholesterol, and most have significant amounts of vitamins A and C, potassium, calcium, iron, other micronutrients and dietary fibre. Also in this category are **eggplant, garlic, leeks, onions and mushrooms** which contain few calories, no cholesterol, and important amounts of potassium, calcium, iron and other micronutrients, as well as dietary fibre. **Red peppers and tomatoes** are low-calorie vegetables with no cholesterol that are loaded with vitamins A and C, iron and dietary fibre. Tomatoes also contain the phytonutrient lycopene. **Avocado and olives** contain some beneficial monounsaturated and polyunsaturated fat, but no cholesterol. Avocados are relatively high in potassium and vitamin A, while olives have significant amounts of iron and calcium.

Grains Group: Includes all foods made from wheat, rice, oats, cornmeal and barley, such as bread, pasta, oatmeal and breakfast cereals. One serving from the grains group consists of approximately 30 grams of bread (one thin slice), or 30 grams of ready-to-eat cereal, or 75 grams of cooked rice, pasta or cooked cereal. At least half of all grains you eat should be whole grains.

Grains are the seeds of varied grasses grown for food. The outermost layer of the grain is an inedible husk, called chaff. The next layer is bran, a protective coating rich in fibre. When this layer is removed, the product is described as pearled or polished. Inside the bran is the endosperm (the starchy part of a grain) and the germ, the part highest in nutrients (e.g., wheat germ). Whole grains have all these components intact. Refined grains have the husk, bran, and germ removed. Many foods are a mixture of whole and refined grains. Check the ingredient list for the words "whole grain" or "whole wheat" to determine if a food is made from a whole grain. (In some countries, to be labeled "whole grain" a food must contain more than 51 percent whole grain by weight.)

Whole grains include: **barley, buckwheat, bulgur, corn, millet, oats, brown rice, rye, wheat and wild rice**. Some whole-grain foods are: **whole-wheat bread, whole-grain ready-to-eat cereal, whole-wheat crackers, oatmeal, popcorn, whole-wheat pasta**, and whole barley (in beef-barley soup). All grains are low in fat and contain no cholesterol. Whole grains are good sources of complex carbohydrates and dietary fibre, as well as several B vitamins (thiamine, riboflavin, niacin, and folate), vitamin E, and minerals (iron, magnesium, and selenium).

Meats, Beans (and nuts) Group: <u>One serving</u> from this group consists of about 30 grams of lean meat, poultry, or fish, or one egg, or 20 grams of shelled seeds, or nuts (including peanut butter), or 30 grams of cooked dry beans. This group can be divided further into the subgroups meat and foul, fish, eggs, beans, and nuts and seeds.

Meat and Foul: **Skinless white-meat chicken and turkey** are relatively low calorie, low fat, low cholesterol foods that are powerful sources of high-quality protein, vitamin B_6, riboflavin, niacin, phosphorus and potassium. Most meats, even **lean meats**, are higher in fat and calories than chicken and turkey, but do provide high-quality protein and some important nutrients such as iron and B-vitamins.

Fish: Most fish are good choices including **cod, halibut, herring, mackerel, salmon, sardines, scallops, shrimp, snapper, trout and tuna.** Nearly all fish contain high levels of essential-fatty acids. (Oily cold-water fish such as wild salmon, sardines, herring, mackerel and tuna are high in omega-3 essential fatty acid. Trout also has comparatively high omega-3 content.) All fish are relatively low-calorie foods and are good sources of the fat-soluble vitamins A and D. (Fish-liver oils have high levels of fat soluble vitamins, and have been used as dietary supplements for many years.) Nutritionally, seafood is better known for its dietary minerals than for its vitamins. This is because some minerals in fish, such as iodine and selenium, are not available at the same levels in most other non-marine foods. Fish are also a good source of iron and potassium. There is, however, a downside to eating fish. Some fish are contaminated with mercury, PCBs, dioxins and other environmental pollutants.

Mercury is a toxic heavy metal that can accumulate in certain fish species. Large predatory fish such as shark, swordfish, king mackerel and tilefish have the highest concentration of mercury and other contaminates. Canned white albacore tuna, a commonly eaten fish, contains higher levels of mercury than canned light tuna. The U.S. Food and Drug Administration advises adults to eat no more than six ounces of high-mercury fish per week.

PCBs are potential human carcinogens that find their way into fresh waters and oceans where they are absorbed by fish. A recent study reported that PCB levels in farmed salmon, especially those in Europe, were about seven times higher than in wild salmon.

For further information about the safety of fish caught locally, contact your local health department. If no advice is available, eat no more than 170 grams per week of fish you have caught from local waters and do not consume any other fish that week.

According to the University of Michigan Integrative Medicine Department, pregnant and nursing women, and young children, should avoid shark, swordfish, king mackerel and tilefish, and strictly limit the amount of other contaminated fish consumed.

Eggs: Current dietary guidelines and the latest research concerning egg consumption appear to be at odds. On the one hand, because a typical egg yoke contains saturated fat and 300 mg of cholesterol, the latest dietary guidelines recommend that egg yolks and whole eggs can be used in moderation (up to one egg per day), but that egg whites and egg substitutes can be used freely since they contain no cholesterol and little or no fat.
On the other hand, others argue that if judged as a whole food and not simply as a source of cholesterol, positives such as the fact that eggs are low calorie, are loaded with high-quality protein, are a good source of vitamin E, etcetera, are apparent. Moreover, researchers at the Harvard Medical School studied egg consumption among 120,000 nurses and other health professionals with normal cholesterol levels and reported no link between eating eggs and heart disease or stroke.

Some medical researchers advise that, if you are at low risk (i.e., you do not smoke, you exercise regularly, you eat a healthy diet and have no family history of heart disease or stroke) and choose to begin eating eggs, you should have a blood test four to six weeks after you start to determine the impact on your total and LDL cholesterol. Based on the test results, you and your doctor can decide – yes or no to your eating more eggs.

Beans: Among the foods in this important subgroup are **black beans, cannelloni beans, dried peas, fava beans, garbanzo beans, red kidney beans, lentils, lima beans, navy beans, and pinto beans**. All beans are inexpensive, low-fat, plant-protein-rich foods that are good sources of B vitamins, potassium, iron, folate, dietary fibre and important isoflavones phytonutrients.

Nuts and Seeds: This category consists of **almonds, cashews, hazelnuts, peanuts, pecans, pistachio nuts, walnuts, flaxseed, pumpkin seeds, sesame seeds, sunflower seeds**, and others. Because nuts and seeds contain significant amounts of essential-fatty acids, they are comparatively high-calorie foods. Most nuts and seeds have a good amount of dietary fibre, vitamin E, potassium, iron and folate. Almonds, cashews, peanuts, and pine nuts contain a significant quantity of plant protein and essential-fatty acids. Walnuts, flaxseed and pumpkin seeds are important sources of plant-based omega-3 fatty acids.

Soy: The soybean is the most widely grown legume. Healthful soy foods such as **tofu, soy nuts, soymilk, soybean oil, and soy protein** are all made from soybeans. All contain a noteworthy amount of plant-based **complete protein** and omega-3 fatty acid as well as vitamin E, potassium, iron and folate. Soy nuts are also high in dietary fibre.

Soybeans, tofu, and other soy-based foods are an excellent alternative to red meat. But there are some suspected dangers from too much soy. So don't overdo it. The Harvard University School of Public Health recommends two to four servings of soy foods per week as a good goal. Furthermore, they caution adults not to take supplements that contain concentrated soy protein or soy extracts, such as isoflavones.

Milk Group: Includes liquid milk and all products and foods made from milk such yogurt and cheese. (Foods that have little or no calcium such as cream, butter and cream cheese are not in this group.) <u>One serving</u> from the milk group consists of 250 mL of milk or yogurt, or 40 grams of natural cheese, or 60 grams of processed cheese.

Milk, yogurt and natural cheeses are high in calcium and protein. Milk is also often fortified with vitamin D. In addition to calcium and protein, yogurt is a particularly wholesome food providing live active bacteria cultures which promote gastrointestinal health. <u>Most choices in this group should be fat free or low fat.</u>

Oils Group: Includes vegetable oils and foods such as nuts, olives, oily fish, avocados, mayonnaise, soft margarine and some salad dressings. You should limit your intake of saturated fats - that is any fat of animal origin.

The oils group overlaps somewhat with many of the others. Liquid oils, however, are unique to this group. **Corn oil, flaxseed oil, safflower oil, sesame oil, soybean oil and sunflower oil** are polyunsaturated; whereas, **canola oil, olive oil and peanut oil** are monounsaturated. All these oils are high in calories and essential-fatty acids. Essential-fatty acids promote absorption of the fat-soluble vitamins A, D, E, and K. Flaxseed, canola and soybean oil contain omega-3 fatty acids. (Note, when purchasing olive oil, choose an oil that is labelled "extra-virgin" or "virgin." Virgin olive oils are produced from the first pressing of the olives, are unrefined and as a result are more healthful.)

Finally, people like different foods and often food prepared in different ways. Culture, religion, moral beliefs, the cost and availability of food, life experiences, food intolerances, and allergies affect food choices. To make sure you get enough nutrients, use Table 5.5 as a starting point to shape your eating patterns. Select from each major food group, and combine to suit your taste. For instance, if you like Mexican cuisine you might choose tortillas from the grains group and beans from the meat and beans group, whereas those who prefer Asian food might choose rice from the grains group and tofu from the meat and beans group.

➡ Everyone should have a medical check-up before making major changes to their eating patterns. This is particularly important for anyone with medical problems and for women who are pregnant or breast- feeding, all of whom should consult a physician or registered dietician to determine an appropriate dietary pattern.

Vitamin and Mineral Supplements

Even though most adults can get all the vitamins and minerals they need by merely consuming a variety of nutritious foods (from the fruit group, the vegetable group, the grains group, the meat and beans group, the milk group, and the oils group), many physicians recommend a daily multi-vitamin/mineral supplement as a kind of insurance policy.

Be aware that some micronutrients, such as the fat-soluble vitamin A, can be harmful if taken in large quantities. To be safe your multi-vitamin/mineral supplement should contain no more than 100 percent of the recommended dietary allowance (RDA) for each vitamin or mineral. Generally, you don't need the high doses in multi-vitamin/mineral supplements labelled "therapeutic" or "extra-strength." There may be medical reasons for taking larger amounts of a vitamin or mineral than the RDA provides, but check with your doctor first.

For example, a physician may advise a pregnant woman to take an iron supplement, and women who could become pregnant to take folic acid in addition to consuming folate-rich foods to reduce the risk of some serious birth defects. Adults over age 50 and vegetarians who do not eat animal foods may be advised to get their vitamin B_{12} from a supplement or from fortified foods. Older adults and people with little exposure to sunlight may need a vitamin D supplement, and individuals who seldom eat dairy products or other rich sources of calcium may need to take a calcium supplement.

Dietary supplement choices include not only vitamins and minerals, but also herbal products and many other widely available substances. Herbal products, however, usually provide only small amounts of vitamins and minerals and their health value is currently being studied.

Food Container Labels

Today, food packages in many nations are required to list certain nutritional information. The food labels on containers consist of several parts, including information usually on the front panel and frequently nutrition facts on a side or rear panel.

The front panel often indicates if nutrients have been added - for example, "iodized salt" lets you know that iodine has been added, and "enriched pasta" (or "enriched" grain of any type) usually means that thiamine, riboflavin, niacin, iron, and folic acid have been added.

The nutrition facts label (such as that often found on the side of a cereal box) indicates the number of calories and nutrients in a serving. The label allows a consumer to compare similar foods to determine, for instance, which brand of a frozen meal is lower in saturated fat, or which breakfast cereal contains more folic acid, and also to ascertain if a food is high or low in a particular nutrient. The ingredient list on the nutrition facts label typically discloses what is in the food, including any nutrients, fats, or sugars that have been added. Ingredients are usually in descending order by weight; i.e., the most abundant ingredient is listed first.

Energy Value of Foods

In order to plan a diet you must be able to estimate the kcalorie value of foods as well as portion sizes. The nutrition facts label on a food package, listing nutrient content, makes it possible to calculate the number of kcalories in a serving if you know that there are roughly:

	kcal per gram
Carbohydrates	4
Protein	4
Alcohol	7
Fat	9

<u>Example 5.1</u>:   Determine the calories in a 250 mL of whole milk. The label on a container of whole milk indicates that 250 mL has 11 grams of carbohydrate, 8 grams of protein and 9 grams of fat. Therefore, the total calories in 250 mL of whole milk can be determined as follows:

11 grams of carbohydrates x 4 kcalories per gram	=	44
8 grams of protein x 4 kcalories per gram	=	32
9 grams fat x 9 kcalories per gram	=	<u>81</u>
		157 kcal

A sense of the relative "fattening effect" of different foods can be obtained from Table 5.6, "Rank (kcalories per 100 g) of Common Foods," on page 107. The extremes of the chart are represented by water the lowest, which has zero kcalories and fat (lard) the highest at about 900 kcalories per 100 grams. Sugar (a pure carbohydrate) is near the middle of the ranking at 400 kcalories per 100 grams. (Note, protein is also approximately 400 kcalories per 100 grams but there is no pure protein food to rank.) If you appreciate that **all foods are some combination of water, carbohydrate, protein, fat and fibre**, this can lead to a better understanding of why a particular food has the caloric value and rank shown in the table.

Some examples: Watermelon is almost entirely water, with some fibre (zero kcal) and carbohydrate, with no protein or fat, and consequently has a very low 26 Calories per 100 grams value. A grape is again mostly water with some fibre and carbohydrate and according to the chart has only 68 kcalories per 100 grams, but a raisin (a dried grape) is almost entirely carbohydrate and fiber with little water and thus has a value of 290 kcalories per 100 grams – closer to a pure carbohydrate. When a food is not listed in the chart, common sense can often be used to estimate its calorie value; e.g., green beans are not listed, but judging from the ranking of similar foods a value of 20 kcalories per 100 grams seems reasonable. Table 5.6 can also be thought of as a listing of the "calorie density" of foods. As an example, the table illustrates that one kilo of carrots contains about 360 kcalories, or approximately the same number as only 100 grams of sirloin steak. (Note that the numbers in the table are approximate calories per 100 grams of fluid or dry weight.)

Moreover, Table 5.6 in combination with a small weighing scale makes a very useful diet aide - allowing the calorie value of many food portions to be estimated quite accurately. It is a simple mater to weigh a piece of meat or a pancake, or a slice of apple pie, and multiple the weight in grams by the kcalorie value per 100 grams (from table 5.6) and divide by 100 to determine the total number of kcalories. Frequently, the preceding approach will result in more precise calorie values than those obtained from the numbers shown in an ordinary calorie table where the portion size is often ambiguously described.

You Need Fibre in your Diet

Fibre is an important part of a healthy diet. **You need to consume fibre to assist your digestive system**. According to the Harvard University School of Public Health, adequate fibre intake reduces the risk of developing various conditions, including heart disease, diabetes, diverticular disease, and constipation.

Three fibres that are eaten on a regular basis are cellulose, hemicellulose and pectin. Hemicellulose is found in the hulls of different grains like wheat; e.g., wheat bran is hemicellulose. Cellulose is the structural component of plants, and gives vegetables their familiar shape. Pectin is found most often in fruits, is soluble in water but non-digestible, and is usually referred to as "water-soluble fibre." When you eat fibre, in any of its forms, it simply passes straight through, untouched by but aiding your digestive system. Zero calories absorbed! Adults should get a least 20-35 grams of dietary fibre per day. The best sources are fresh fruits and vegetables, nuts and legumes, and whole-grain foods.

Food	kcal	Food	kcal	Food	kcal
Water	**0**	Peas	71	Liverwurst	278
Coffee/Tea	4	Yogurt (whole)	73	Hamburger	286
Vinegar	9	Potato (boiled)	76	Tuna (in oil)	288
Lettuce	15	Clams (raw)	79	Raisins	290
Celery	16	Banana	85	Bologna	304
Asparagus	23	Corn	87	Wheat Flakes	310
Tomato	24	Wine	88	Cake (average)	350
Spinach	25	Lobster	93	Sirloin Steak	360
Watermelon	26	Lentils	106	Cheese	370
Lemon	27	Scallops	112	Ham (baked)	370
Broccoli	28	Rice	114	Oatmeal	375
Mushrooms	30	Beans	118	**Sugar**	**400**
Cantaloupe	30	Pasta	125	Pretzels	390
Milk (fat free)	32	Tuna (in water)	127	Graham Crackers	400
Carrots	36	Olives (black)	129	Doughnut	410
Strawberries	37	Blue Fish (baked)	159	Fudge	410
Green Pepper	37	Egg (boiled)	163	Chocolate	530
Peach	38	Turkey (light meat)	176	Potato Chips	568
Grapefruit	40	Ice Cream	193	Peanut Butter	585
Cola Drink	42	Sardines	196	Almonds	598
Beer	44	Turkey (dark meat)	203	Bacon	611
Yogurt non fat	44	Pancakes	225	Walnuts	630
Orange	50	Bread (wheat)	243	Butter	716
Apple	56	Whisky-86 proof	249	Mayonnaise	718
Milk (whole)	66	Apple Pie	256	Margarine	720
Cherries	68	Bread (white)	270	Vegetable Oil	884
Grapes	68	Jam/Jelly	272	**Lard (fat)**	**900**

Table 5.6: Rank (kcalories per 100 g) of Common Foods

Drink Lots of Water

The average adult female body is about 52 percent water, while the average adult male body is approximately 63 percent water. If you are average, everyday you lose about 2500 mL of water when you breathe, perspire, and excrete waste. Because water is needed for almost every biochemical and physiologic process in your body, to maintain your body's water balance you must replace this lost water. (The water in your body is said to be balanced, when your water intake from all sources equals your loss of water.)

Typically, the food you eat every day contains about 750 mL of mostly concealed water. When you metabolize the food you eat, you create another 250 mL of water. That leaves about 1500 mL that must be replaced by the liquids you drink – more when you exercise. It appears, therefore, that the long-established wisdom advocating that you drink eight glasses of water per day (or any healthy beverage such as fruit juice) is close to the mark.

Go Easy on Salt

Sodium and sodium chloride (salt) normally occur in small quantities in many natural foods. Salt and sodium-containing ingredients are also frequently found in high amounts in processed foods, such as canned soup and baked goods. People also add salt during food preparation and to the food they eat.

Although sodium plays an important role in your body, many studies have demonstrated that high sodium intake is also associated with high blood pressure. In your body, sodium retains water expanding blood volume which in turn raises blood pressure. Moreover, although some questions remain, evidence suggests that many adults who are predisposed to high blood pressure (for example having a parent who has high blood pressure) can reduce their chances of developing high blood pressure by consuming less sodium.

Most people consume too much sodium. The U.S. Department of Health and Human Services recommends that healthy adults **limit sodium intake to 2,400 mg per day.** (Note that five millilitres of salt contain about 2,300 mg of sodium.) Of course, individuals who have high blood pressure and are salt sensitive are often advised to limit their sodium intake even further.

Restrict Your Use of Sugar

Sugars are carbohydrates and come in many forms. Sugar is found naturally in fruits, some vegetables, milk, breads, cereals and grains, and is often added to foods during processing, preparation and when eating. Added sugar and naturally occurring sugars are chemically identical and your body cannot distinguish between them.

Cake, cookies, candy and many beverages contain large amounts of added sugar that supply a large number of "nutritionally-empty calories." Only very active people with high calorie needs can afford to consume any quantity of these sugar-laden foods. **Sugar should be used sparingly** by people with low calorie needs and in moderation by most other healthy adults. (Contrary to what many believe, the latest scientific evidence seems to indicate diets high in sugar do not cause diabetes. Rather, scientific evidence indicates that adult-onset diabetes occurs most often in those who are overweight.)

Limit Alcohol & Caffeine

Wine and beer contain a small amount of nutrients and micronutrients, but other alcoholic beverages, such as whiskey, vodka and gin consist of nothing but "nutritionally-empty calories." Because alcohol has effects that can also be harmful when consumed in excess, it is worth repeating: If you drink alcohol do so in moderation.

Some research has shown that moderate drinking is associated with a lower risk of coronary- heart disease, but high levels of alcohol intake also raise your risk for high blood pressure, stroke, heart disease, certain cancers, birth defects, and of course accidents. Heavy drinking may cause cirrhosis of the liver, inflammation of the pancreas, brain damage, and in some cases malnutrition (because alcohol contains calories that are often substituted for those in more nutritious foods).

Caffeine should also be used in moderation. Caffeine is found in coffee, tea, some soft drinks and foods that contain cocoa. It is also in some drugs such as cold remedies and in medicine sold over the counter to relieve headaches.

About Sports Drinks

When you sweat, you lose both water and salt. An imbalance of any of the electrolytes in your body (such as sodium) can be harmful and even dangerous. You can make sure you're replacing the sodium you lose when you sweat during exercise by consuming a sports drink - and many endurance athletes do just that when participating in long events.

But this ebook is not for endurance athletes, it is a guide for those of us who typically workout moderately for an hour or less. In fact, the majority of exercise physiologists feel that sports drinks are unnecessary for most people, and that plain water, along with the salt in the food we eat, are all that is needed to replenish the water and sodium lost during moderate exercise.

Common Sense Nutrition

- **Know your daily caloric allowance** whether you are trying to maintain your weight or are on a reducing diet. (We will cover this in detail in Chapter 6, "Weight Control" that follows immediately.)

- **Eat a variety of foods** within your caloric allowance, and use Table 5.5 to shape your eating patterns. Try to choose the proper quantity from each food group.

- **Try not to consume foods containing partially-hydrogenated vegetable oil** because they are high in trans fats. This includes commercially prepared baked goods, snack foods, and processed foods, including fast foods.

- **Limit your intake of saturated fats.** Eat meat less often and fish and poultry more often, and use fat-free milk and milk products.

- **When possible, select fresh and natural foods and whole-grain products,** and avoid chemical preservatives and additives, artificial and imitation foods, refined and processed foods, and foods that are comprised of "nutritionally-empty calories."

- **Eat nutritionally-dense foods** rather than calorie-dense foods.

- Before you buy, **read and understand the labels on food packages.**

One final point, try to **eat slowly.** If you are someone who eats fast, who finishes before everyone else at the table, you are not giving yourself a chance to feel full. While everyone else is still eating, you either sit there and pick, or you have seconds, taking in extra calories you could avoid if you would just slow down. To slow down, try talking more at the table, and try chewing your food more thoroughly.

6. WEIGHT CONTROL

Obesity and overweight are major public health problems. Obesity raises the risk of heart disease, some cancers, diabetes and arthritis, and being overweight often elevates blood pressure and cholesterol, which in turn can increase the risk of heart disease.

Because obesity and overweight are so common and public interest is so great, we are all continually assaulted by a blinding array of fad diets, miracle pills, health spas, exercise devices, reducing belts, and the like. Most people are left bewildered not knowing what to believe. The truth is that weight control, although a relatively complex issue, is governed by a set of logical, scientific principles, and the acceptance and understanding of these principles – augmented of course by desire and self-discipline – can lead you to sure and lasting weight management.

Causes of Overweight & Obesity

Before starting, it is important to have an understanding of the causes of overweight and obesity. The popular notion that most people are overweight or obese because of a defect in their metabolism is just not supported by scientific evidence. In fact, being overweight or obese most often can be attributed to how we adapt to our 21st century environment and to our heredity. More specifically, the major causes of obesity and overweight are as follows:

- **Environmental**: We live in a society where food is abundant and where strenuous physical activity is, for most people, a thing of the past. In other words, we eat too much and do too little. This is by far the most important factor.

- **Genetic**: Everyone starts life with a different body type. Researchers agree there is a relationship between the body type we inherit and the likelihood and ease with which we become overweight. Three basic body types are illustrated in Figure 6.1 on the next page. The active ectomorph, with a typically long, narrow body and light appetite will find it difficult indeed to gain weight or to become overweight. On the other extreme, the more sedentary endomorph with a hearty appetite faces a life-long struggle against obesity. Depending on their appetite and how active they are, even muscular mesomorphs often gain unwanted weight as they age. Because everyone has some features of each body type, we are all born with different weight gaining tendencies.

- **Psychological**: There are a great many people who overeat and become overweight in response to tension, frustration, or other psychological issues.

- **Developmental**: Early forced feeding often leads to childhood-onset obesity. Overeating then becomes habitual and an excessive number of fat cells are formed early on that are difficult to shed later in life.

- **Metabolic and Regulatory**: Sometimes overeating is caused by a damaged hypothalamus or an incorrect interpretation of the hunger/satiety signal. Though relatively rare, a defect in the thyroid or pituitary gland can also cause a change in metabolic rate. All can result in overweight.

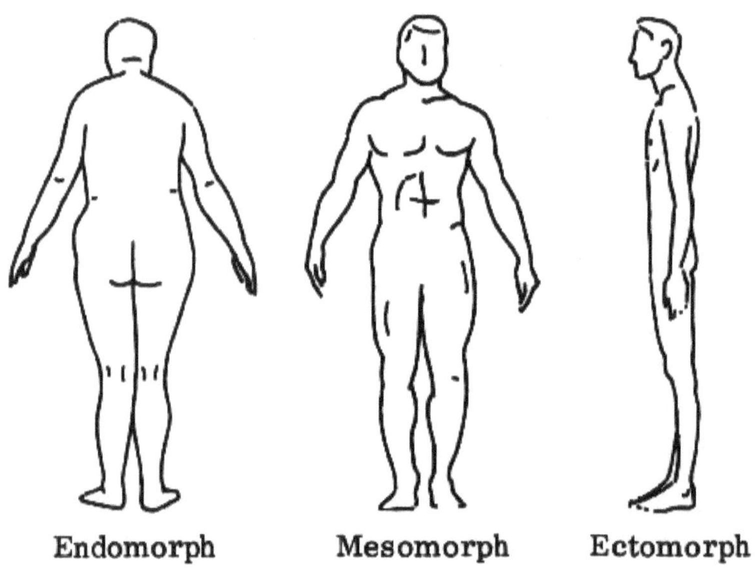

Figure 6.1: Human Body Types
We are in the process of substituting female for the male figures.

The net result of all of the preceding is that hundreds of millions of people all over the world are overweight or obese, carrying unhealthy, unattractive, excess poundage.

Weight Change and Energy

Our bodies use energy, called basal metabolic energy, just to remain alive – for breathing, for maintenance of muscle tone, etcetera. We use additional energy when we carry out the physical activities of daily living – when we sit, stand, work, walk, run. As illustrated in Figure 6.2 (on page 113), the total amount of energy we expend everyday is the sum of the basal energy and the energy expended in physical activity. Our energy source is the food we eat minus waste.

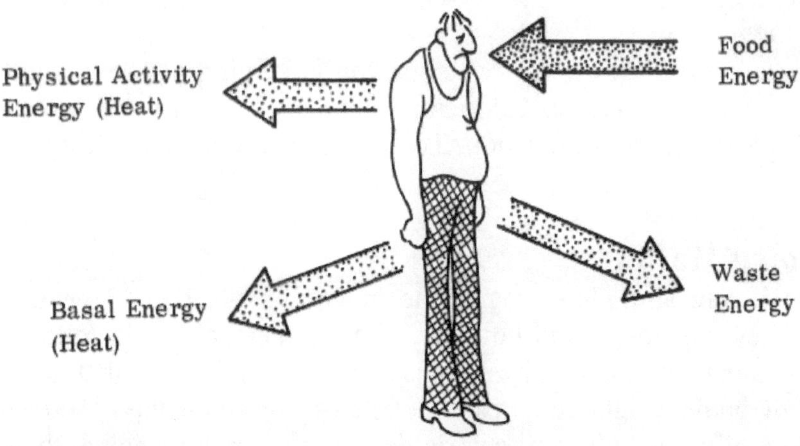

Figure 6.2: Forms of Energy Intake & Expended by the Humans
We are in the process of substituting female for the male figures.

According to the well established, scientifically valid, conservation of energy principle, when the human body is in energy equilibrium, the energy value of the food consumed minus waste, equals the sum of the basal energy and the energy expended during physical activity. When the energy taken in equals the total energy expended, weight is neither gained nor lost. When there is an energy imbalance, however, weight is either gained or lost. In general we can state:

- **WEIGHT GAIN occurs when your food energy intake is greater than the total energy you expend. In this case your body stores the extra energy as fat.**

- **WEIGHT LOSS occurs when your food energy intake is less than the total energy you expend. In this case your body converts stored fat (and in some cases muscle) into energy.**

The measure of energy, whether in the form of food, physical activity, or heat is the calorie. As mentioned previously, weight loss occurs when you eat fewer calories than the total calories you use in daily living. This difference in calories is referred to as the calorie deficit. How much weight you lose depends on the magnitude of the calorie deficit. In technical terms, the **calorie deficit, or calorie difference, is the driving force for weight change**. (The scientifically astute will appreciate that the calorie deficit which is the driving force for weight change is somewhat analogous to the voltage difference which is the driving force for the flow of electricity, and to a temperature difference which is the driving force for the flow of heat.)

Researchers have shown that whether you are trying to lose weight or just maintain your weight, it is calories that count. In theory it does not matter what foods the calories are from. Too much of any food can result in weight gain.

Slimming Math

People on any slimming programme invariably want to know how much weight they will lose - and how fast. Simple metabolic calculations make a rough estimate possible. Physiologists have long known that to lose one pound of body weight requires a deficit of approximately 3500 kcalories. Therefore, if a person's total calorie deficit over time is known, their weight loss over time can be calculated. As will be evident in a later section, "Keeping It Off," a relatively inactive 30 year-old woman weighing a few pounds less than 11 st 5lbs expends about 2500 kcalories in day-to-day living. (In other words, if this woman eats about 2500 kcalories per day she will neither gain nor lose weight.) If she goes on a 1500 kcalorie per day slimming diet, her daily deficit would be 2500 – 1500 = 1000 kcalories. In one week her deficit would be 1000 kcalories per day x 7 days = 7000 kcalories, and she should lose 7000 / 3500, or two pounds.

This computation technique, however, is somewhat crude. Primarily because the preceding calculation does not account for a very important scientific fact: As we lose weight we actually need fewer calories to maintain our lower weight. As a result, if a dieter's calorie intake remains constant over some period of time, their calorie deficit will decrease during their diet and the rate at which they lose weight will also decrease with time.

Weight Loss Prediction Tables

Fortunately, a more precise determination of the rate of weight loss is possible. Scientists have long known that **weight loss is a function of age, sex, height, weight, physical activity, caloric intake and the duration of the diet (or time on the diet)**. This writer related all these variables in a complex, scientifically based, energy-weight-control equation, published in the *American Journal of Clinical Nutrition*, and subsequently published a set of 60 Weight Loss Prediction tables. In this edition of *Total Fitness* you will find an abridged set of six Weight Loss Prediction tables (Tables 6.2 through 6.7, on pages 117 to 122).

Selecting the Correct Weight Loss Prediction Table

Your first task is to choose the correct Weight Loss Prediction table. The twelve Weight Loss Prediction tables are organized by gender, age and activity level. Only two activity levels are covered in this text:

1) <u>Relatively Inactive During and after Work</u>: This is self-explanatory. It applies to individuals who sit at a desk most of the day and engage in no after hours exercise.

2) <u>Moderately Active During or After Work</u>: To qualify for this category, you would have to either have a physically strenuous job (such as a construction worker, postal worker delivering mail on foot, etcetera), or engage in some form of regular exercise everyday after work (e.g., taking a brisk three-mile walk, working out in a gym, and so forth).

Use Table 6.1 to find the Weight Loss Prediction Table that is right for you:

Gender	Age	Activity Level	Table No.	Go to Page
Females	18 – 35	Relatively inactive	6.2	117
	18 - 35	Moderately active	6.3	118
	36 - 55	Relatively inactive	6.4	119
	36 - 55	Moderately active	6.5	120
	56 - 75	Relatively inactive	6.6	121
	56 - 75	Moderately active	6.7	122

Table 6.1: Selecting the Correct Weight Loss Prediction Table

Weight Loss Prediction Example

Example 6.1: A 40-year-old woman, who weighs 13 stone, has essentially a sedentary job as a computer programmer and spends most of her free time in front of a TV set. How long will it take her to lose 2 stone?

First she should choose Table 6.4 (on page 119), labelled "Weight Loss Prediction for Relatively Inactive Women, Ages 36 - 55 years." Then she should scan the far left of the table and locate her present weight of 13 stone; from this number she would move a finger horizontally (to the right) until it intersects the vertical column headed by the 2 stone weight loss she desires. The three numbers at the intersection are the time in days for her to lose weight, depending on the diet kcalories consumed. Specifically, to lose 3 stone our fictional female's calorie intake options are:

- 900 kcalories per day for 70 days.

- 1200 kcalories per day for 87 days.

- 1500 kcalories per day for 115 days.

Which alternative should she choose? Health professionals recommend a gradual weight loss of two pounds per week. In this case, her diet should last about fourteen weeks, or 98 days, pointing to either the 1200 kcal or 1500 kcal diet options.

Please note that the calorie allowance during a weight loss diet need not be the same for every day of the week. It is the average intake over the entire week that counts.

WEIGHT LOSS PREDICTION FOR WOMEN 18 - 35.
(Relatively Inactive During and After Working Hours)

Weight (Stone)	Diet kcal	Weight Loss Desired (Stone)							
		0.5	1.0	1.5	2.0	2.5	3.0	3.5	4.0
9.0	900	22	45	70					
	1200	29	60	95					
	1500	43	91	146					
10.0	900	20	41	62	86				
	1200	25	52	81	113				
	1500	35	73	116	164				
11.0	900	18	37	56	77	99	123		
	1200	22	46	71	98	127	159		
	1500	30	62	97	135	178	226		
12.0	900	17	34	52	70	90	111	133	156
	1200	20	41	64	88	113	140	169	200
	1500	26	54	83	115	150	189	231	279
13.0	900	15	31	48	65	83	102	121	142
	1200	18	38	58	79	101	125	150	177
	1500	23	48	74	101	131	163	198	236
14.0	900	14	29	44	60	77	94	112	131
	1200	17	35	53	72	92	114	136	160
	1500	21	43	66	90	116	144	174	206
15.0	1200	16	32	49	67	85	104	125	146
	1500	19	39	60	82	105	129	155	183
	1800	24	50	77	106	137	170	207	246
16.0	1200	15	30	46	62	79	97	115	134
	1500	18	36	55	75	96	118	141	165
	1800	22	45	69	94	121	150	181	215
17.0	1200	14	28	43	58	74	90	107	125
	1500	16	33	51	69	88	108	129	151
	1800	20	41	62	85	109	135	162	191

Numbers in table indicate time in days to obtain desired weight loss.

Table 6.2:   Weight Loss Prediction for Relatively Inactive Women, 18 – 35

WEIGHT LOSS PREDICTION FOR WOMEN 18 - 35.
(Moderately Active During or After Working Hours)

Weight (Stone)	Diet kcal	Weight Loss Desired (Stone)							
		0.5	1.0	1.5	2.0	2.5	3.0	3.5	4.0
9.0	900	19	39	61					
	1200	24	50	78		Numbers in table indicate time in days to obtain desired weight loss.			
	1500	33	69	110					
10.0	900	17	35	54	74				
	1200	21	43	67	93				
	1500	27	57	90	126				
11.0	900	16	32	49	67	86	105		
	1200	19	38	59	82	106	132		
	1500	24	49	76	106	139	175		
12.0	900	14	29	45	61	78	96	115	135
	1200	17	35	53	73	94	117	141	166
	1500	21	43	66	92	119	149	181	218
13.0	900	13	27	41	56	72	88	105	123
	1200	15	32	49	66	85	105	126	148
	1500	19	38	59	81	105	130	157	187
14.0	900	12	25	38	52	66	81	97	113
	1200	14	29	45	61	78	95	114	134
	1500	17	35	53	73	94	116	139	165
15.0	1200	13	27	41	56	71	88	105	122
	1500	15	32	49	66	85	105	125	147
	1800	19	38	59	81	105	130	157	186
16.0	1200	12	25	38	52	66	81	97	113
	1500	14	29	45	61	78	95	114	134
	1800	17	35	53	73	94	116	139	164
17.0	1200	12	24	36	49	62	76	90	105
	1500	13	27	41	56	72	88	105	123
	1800	16	32	49	67	85	105	126	148

Table 6.3: Weight Loss Prediction for Moderately Active Women, 18 – 35

WEIGHT LOSS PREDICTION FOR WOMEN 36 - 55.
(Relatively Inactive During and After Working Hours)

Weight (Stone)	Diet kcal	Weight Loss Desired (Stone)							
		0.5	1.0	1.5	2.0	2.5	3.0	3.5	4.0
9.0	900	24	50	78					
	1200	33	69	109					
	1500	52	111	182					
10.0	900	22	44	69	94				
	1200	28	59	92	128				
	1500	41	87	139	198				
11.0	900	20	40	62	84	109	134		
	1200	25	51	80	110	143	179		
	1500	34	72	113	159	211	270		
12.0	900	18	37	56	77	98	121	145	171
	1200	22	46	71	97	126	156	189	225
	1500	30	61	96	133	174	220	272	332
13.0	900	17	34	52	70	90	110	132	155
	1200	20	41	64	87	112	139	167	197
	1500	26	54	83	115	149	187	228	274
14.0	900	15	31	48	65	83	102	121	142
	1200	19	38	58	79	102	125	150	177
	1500	23	48	74	102	131	163	197	235
15.0	1200	17	35	54	73	93	114	137	160
	1500	21	43	67	91	117	145	175	206
	1800	28	57	88	122	159	199	242	291
16.0	1200	16	32	50	67	86	105	126	147
	1500	19	40	61	83	106	131	157	185
	1800	25	51	78	108	139	173	209	249
17.0	1200	15	30	46	63	80	98	116	136
	1500	18	36	56	76	97	119	143	167
	1800	22	46	70	96	124	153	185	218

Numbers in table indicate time in days to obtain desired weight loss.

Table 6.4: Weight Loss Prediction for Relatively Inactive Women, 36 – 55

WEIGHT LOSS PREDICTION FOR WOMEN 36 - 55.

(Moderately Active During or After Working Hours)

Weight (Stone)	Diet kcal	Weight Loss Desired (Stone)							
		0.5	1.0	1.5	2.0	2.5	3.0	3.5	4.0
9.0	900	21	43	66					
	1200	27	56	87					
	1500	38	80	129					
10.0	900	18	38	58	80				
	1200	23	48	75	103				
	1500	31	65	103	145				
11.0	900	17	34	53	72	93	115		
	1200	20	42	65	90	117	146		
	1500	26	55	86	120	158	200		
12.0	900	15	31	48	65	84	103	124	146
	1200	18	38	58	80	103	128	154	183
	1500	23	48	74	103	134	168	205	248
13.0	900	14	29	44	60	77	94	113	132
	1200	17	34	53	72	92	114	137	162
	1500	20	42	65	90	116	145	176	210
14.0	900	13	27	41	56	71	87	103	121
	1200	15	31	48	66	84	103	124	145
	1500	18	38	58	80	103	128	154	183
15.0	1200	14	29	44	60	77	95	113	132
	1500	17	34	53	72	93	115	138	162
	1800	21	43	66	91	117	145	176	210
16.0	1200	13	27	41	56	71	87	104	121
	1500	16	32	49	67	85	104	125	146
	1800	19	38	59	81	104	129	155	184
17.0	1200	12	25	38	52	66	81	96	112
	1500	14	29	45	61	78	95	114	133
	1800	17	35	54	73	94	116	139	164

Numbers in table indicate time in days to obtain desired weight loss.

Table 6.5:   Weight Loss Prediction for Moderately Active Women, 36 – 55

WEIGHT LOSS PREDICTION FOR WOMEN 56 - 75.
(Relatively Inactive During and After Working Hours)

Weight (Stone)	Diet kcal	Weight Loss Desired (Stone)							
		0.5	1.0	1.5	2.0	2.5	3.0	3.5	4.0
9.0	900	26	54	84					
	1200	37	77	121					
	1500	61	133	222					
10.0	900	23	48	74	102				
	1200	31	65	101	141				
	1500	47	101	162	234				
11.0	900	21	43	66	90	117	144		
	1200	27	56	87	121	157	197		
	1500	39	81	129	182	243	315		
12.0	900	19	39	60	82	105	129	156	183
	1200	24	50	77	106	137	170	207	247
	1500	33	68	107	150	197	250	311	
13.0	900	18	36	55	75	96	118	141	165
	1200	22	45	69	94	121	150	182	215
	1500	29	59	92	128	166	209	256	310
14.0	900	16	33	51	69	88	108	129	151
	1200	20	41	62	85	110	135	162	191
	1500	25	52	81	112	145	180	219	261
15.0	1200	18	37	57	78	101	123	147	172
	1500	23	47	73	100	128	159	192	227
	1800	31	64	99	137	179	226	277	336
16.0	1200	17	35	53	72	92	113	135	157
	1500	21	43	66	90	115	142	171	202
	1800	27	56	87	120	155	194	235	282
17.0	1200	16	32	49	67	85	104	124	145
	1500	19	39	60	82	105	129	155	182
	1800	24	50	77	106	137	170	205	244

Numbers in table indicate time in days to obtain desired weight loss.

Table 6.6: Weight Loss Prediction for Relatively Inactive Women, 56 – 75

WEIGHT LOSS PREDICTION FOR WOMEN 56 - 75
(Moderately Active During or After Working Hours)

Weight (Stone)	Diet kcal	Weight Loss Desired (Stone)							
		0.5	1.0	1.5	2.0	2.5	3.0	3.5	4.0
9.0	900	22	45	71					
	1200	29	61	95		Numbers in table indicate time in days to obtain desired weight loss.			
	1500	43	91	148					
10.0	900	20	40	62	86				
	1200	25	52	81	112				
	1500	34	72	115	163				
11.0	900	18	36	56	76	98	122		
	1200	22	45	70	97	126	157		
	1500	29	60	95	133	175	224		
12.0	900	16	33	51	69	89	109	131	155
	1200	20	40	62	85	110	137	166	198
	1500	25	52	81	112	146	184	227	276
13.0	900	15	30	46	63	81	99	119	140
	1200	18	36	56	77	99	122	147	174
	1500	22	46	71	97	126	158	192	230
14.0	900	14	28	43	58	75	91	109	128
	1200	16	33	51	70	89	110	132	155
	1500	20	41	63	86	111	138	167	198
15.0	1200	15	31	47	64	82	100	120	141
	1500	18	37	57	78	100	124	148	175
	1800	23	46	72	99	128	159	194	232
16.0	1200	14	28	43	59	75	92	110	129
	1500	16	34	52	71	90	111	133	157
	1800	20	41	64	88	113	140	169	201
17.0	1200	13	27	40	55	70	86	102	119
	1500	15	31	48	65	83	102	121	142
	1800	18	37	58	79	101	125	150	178

Table 6.7: Weight Loss Prediction for Moderately Active Women, 56 – 75

Your Weight Loss Rate Will Decrease Over Time

It is well known that if your caloric intake on a slimming diet is constant, your rate of weight loss will decrease with time. In other words, as you lose weight it will get more difficult, or rather it will take a longer time to lose additional weight!

Let's consider the woman in Example 1 (page 116). To understand this decreasing weight loss rate we have to jump ahead to Weight Maintenance Table 6.19, on page 133. (The weight maintenance tables list how many calories you can eat to neither gain nor lose weight.)

Recall that a calorie deficit is the driving force for weight loss. A person's calorie deficit is determined by subtracting diet calorie from the maintenance calories. The amount of weight lost in a week is equal to kcal deficit times 7 divided by 3500.

From Table 6.19 we find that before she began her diet, she must have been consuming about 2550 kcalories per day to maintain her weight at 13 stone. At the start of her 1200-kcalorie diet, therefore, her deficit was 2550 − 1200 = 1350 kcalories per day, and she would have started losing weight at a rate of (1350 x 7/3500), about 2.7 pounds per week. At the end of her diet, the same table shows that at 11 stone she would have to eat no more than 2302 kcalories per day to neither gain nor lose weight. Her deficit would have been only 2302 − 1200 = 1102 kcalories per day, and her weight lose rate would have dropped to (1102 x 7/3500), 2.2 pounds per week.

Weight Change Due to Water Variations

When there is a calorie deficit the resulting weight loss is variable in its composition. Fat, water and protein (muscle, bone mass, etcetera) are lost at different rates at different times in the diet. Because water is often a significant component of weight loss, it is essential to understand how the amount of water in your body varies.

First, **realize that your body weight fluctuates about two pounds daily – whether on a diet or not**. Your weight is lowest in the morning before breakfast and highest in the evening before retiring. In addition, the quantity of water in your body also varies from day to day. Over a reasonable period of time, however, it can be stated that the amount of fluid leaving your body will equal the amount entering your body by way of food and drink. The water balance of your body is then said to be in equilibrium.

At the start of any diet, there is usually a considerable loss of body water, and since 500 mL of water weighs about one pound this initial water loss will appear to be a weight loss. But this weight loss is not "real" because only a small quantity of body tissue has been lost. (Many theories have been proposed to explain this phenomenon but none have been scientifically confirmed.) Changes in body hydration, therefore, cause higher weight loss during the first week or two of a diet than is shown in the Weight Loss Prediction tables. By the following week, however, the body's water balance will again readjust and the total weight loss should more closely approach the values in the tables.

The Weight Loss Plateau

Many slimmers complain that after losing some amount of weight, they are stuck; they reach a so-called "plateau," and stop losing weight – at least for some time period. If this happens to you, you will probably get discouraged and frustrated and wonder what you should do to break through and start losing weight again. Before we address solutions, let us examine the possible causes of a weight loss plateau.

First, you could actually still be losing weight but at such a such low a rate that your weight loss is masked by the natural daily fluctuations in your weight, and your perception is that you have reached a plateau. The low weight loss rate is no doubt due to the much lower calorie deficit associated with your new lower weight - as described in the previous section "Your Weight Loss Rate Will Decreases Over Time." Recall, as you lose weight it gets increasingly harder to lose additional weight. If this is the case, the solution is to increase your calorie deficit by either reducing your caloric intake or increasing your activity level – or both. This done you should once more see a more detectable weight loss each week.

The most probable cause for a real weight loss plateau, however, is that over time you have become careless, either eating slightly more, or exercising less, or both. Yet another cause could be temporary water retention as discussed in the preceding section. More than likely it is a combination of all of these factors that makes you believe you have stopped losing weight.

If you encounter a weight loss plateau, the first thing to do is sit back and analyze your eating and exercise patterns. A good technique is to keep a diet diary, honestly listing everything you eat and the associated calories. (Most people underestimate their caloric intake by about 15 percent.) Add the calories consumed for a week and divide by seven to compute an average daily caloric intake. Then enter either Table 6.19 (on page 133) at your current weight and activity level and determine your maintenance calories. Next, calculate your all-important daily caloric deficit (maintenance calories minus your daily caloric intake). Then make an estimate of your expected weekly weight loss by multiplying your daily caloric deficit by seven and dividing the result by 3500. Consider the example that follows.

Weight Loss Plateau Example

Example 6.2: A relatively inactive 60-year-old woman, who weighed 14 st 7lb and is on a 1500 kcalorie slimming diet. She reached 9st 7lb, but feels she has stopped losing weight, has reached a plateau. How should she proceed?

First, she conducts a careful review of her eating patterns and finds that her average daily intake is not 1500 kcalories but is actually closer to 1800 kcalories. Again we jump ahead to Weight Maintenance Table 6.19 (on page 133) where she determines that at 9st 7lb her weight maintenance calorie level is about 2024 kcalories per day. Her daily deficit then is only 2024 – 1800 = 224 kcalories. In one week she will lose a meagre 224 x 7 / 3500 = 0.45 pounds, less than half a pound per week!

So she is probably still losing weight, albeit so slowly that in the short term her assessment is that her weight loss has stopped and she has hit a mysterious weight loss blocking plateau. As a rule then, to avoid the perception that a dreaded weight loss plateau has been reached, you should not allow your deficit to fall below 500 kcalories per day. This will assure a more observable weight loss of at least one pound per week.

Slimming Principles

Once the parameters involved in slimming are related in a mathematical equation, it is possible to state some principles or maxims. (It is also possible to deduce the following truisms by examining the Weight Loss Prediction tables.)

- Given two people the same age, gender and activity level, and on the same reducing diet, **the heavier person will lose weight faster than the thinner person**. For example, according to Table 6.4 on page 119, on 1500 kcalories, it would take a relatively inactive 50 year old female weighing 10 stone 71 days to lose one stone; whereas the same table indicates a female weighing 20 stone would only take 27 days to lose one stone.

- Given a male and female, the same age, weight, activity level and on the same reducing diet (i.e., consuming the same number of calories), **the man will lose weight faster than the woman**. This is due to the fact that women have lower basal metabolic rates than men and therefore must eat less than a man to lose the same amount of weight.

- Given two individuals, the same gender, weight and activity level, **the younger person will lose weight faster than the older person.** The lesson is if you are overweight start on a weight-loss diet now because it will become **more difficult to lose weight as you get older.**

- It follows that if your **caloric intake is constant over the years you will slowly gain weight as you age.** This is because your basal metabolic rate decreases as you advance in age, and most people tend not to be as active as they get older.

- If your **caloric intake on a slimming diet is constant, your rate of weight loss will decrease with time**. As noted earlier, as you lose weight it gets more difficult, or rather it takes more time to lose the next half stone.

Slimming Diets

Sure you want to lose weight but which slimming diet should you choose? Low carb, high protein, low fat? Atkins, Zone, South Beach, Pritikin, or Ornish? What about the grapefruit diet or Sugar Busters? And on and on. Each fad diet that comes along promises to be the true path to weight loss.

In reality you can lose weight on almost any diet. Many of the aforementioned diets don't even mention the word calorie, but when carefully scrutinized it is clear that by restricting certain foods these diets are in fact limiting calories. You lose weight when you eat fewer calories than your body burns. It doesn't matter whether the calories are from protein, carbohydrates or fat. Calories are calories.

Low-fat diets gained popularity in the 1990's. And you can lose weight on a low-fat diet provided you also lower your calorie intake. But in recent years, even the firmest fat-limiting advocates have to admit that not all fats are alike. Some fats are bad for you, but others are actually healthy and should be included in any diet – including a weight-loss diet.

Anecdotal evidence and weight-loss research indicates that early on you will probably lose weight faster on a low-carb diet. The reason is two-fold. First at the start of any diet there is usually considerable loss of water – and water loss is particularly high for low-carb diets. But the main reason is that when you exclude carbohydrate-rich foods, you have no choice but to eat more fats and protein. Because fats and protein are digested more slowly than carbohydrates, most people don't feel quite as hungry on a low-carb reducing diet. So they eat less – eat fewer calories overall – and lose weight. The problem with low-carb diets is that they are nutritionally unsound and are difficult to stay with over the long haul. So what to do?

What Makes a Good Slimming Diet?

Every good slimming diet must have the following three characteristics:

1) **A good slimming diet must provide you with an understanding of weight control as well as the knowledge you need to reduce your weight to the desired level.**

2) **A good slimming diet must help you remain healthy while you are losing weight.**

3) **A good slimming diet must lead you to a healthier way of eating and exercising that will help you keep off the weight you have lost.**

The slimming diet that fits these constraints is the so-called "balanced diet; " i.e., a diet that is not only low calorie but also nutritionally balanced and complies with the guidelines set forth in Table 5.5 (on page 98).

Planning Slimming Eating Patterns

Using the information presented to this point, you should be able to plan a slimming diet suited to your individual likes and lifestyle. This offers great flexibility, but requires that you take care and use Table 5.5 as a guide in choosing foods from all six-food groups.

After you determine your daily diet calorie allowance from the Weight Loss Prediction Tables, the next step is to decide on a weekly routine, i.e., how you plan to distribute your calories among the days of the week. As already mentioned your calorie allowance need not be the same for every day of the week. Next apportion your daily caloric allowance among the meals of the day according to your personal eating habits. This writer recommends the following approximate daily calorie distribution.

Daily kcalorie Distribution

	900	1200	1500	1800
Breakfast	200	200	250	250
Mid-day Meal	250	250	350	420
Evening Meal	450	670	780	940
Elective	0	80	150	190

Despite all the information that has been provided here, if you would rather not go through the trouble of planning a personal diet routine, consult a registered dietician. Registered dieticians translate the science of nutrition into everyday information about food, and are trained to assist people with their individual diets and meal plans. Go online to find a registered dietician in your area.

Exchanging Foods: To prevent a diet from becoming monotonous, after about a month, try exchanging or substituting foods – a technique used by dieticians. Exchanging a food listed in a diet for another food with approximately equal caloric value and nutritional content is the foundation of a successful long-term diet. Substitution possibilities are almost endless but have to be done carefully. The easiest substitutions are those within the same food group, such as exchanging one vegetable variety for another, or a glass of milk for an equal amount of yogurt. More sophisticated exchanges cross food groups, for instance replacing 115 grams of lean meat with a tablespoon of peanut butter spread on a piece of whole-wheat bread. Both foods are complete protein and both contain about 170 kcalories.

When on a diet **simple is better** – because the meals you prepare then contain fewer "hidden calories." For example, straightforward broiled fish with microwave vegetables makes a nutritious, quick, low-calorie meal. Lastly, do acquire a good low-calorie cookbook. Be sure the recipes cover breakfast, mid-day and evening meals, and all the recipes contain nutritional information, especially the number of calories per serving. Also obtain a comprehensive food calorie guide such as the excellent U.S. D. A. Home and Garden Bulletin No. 72: "Nutritive Value of Foods." Download at no cost.

Set Meals & Calorie Control

Are you concerned about having to count calories? Whether on a reducing diet or trying to maintain your weight, allocating a specific number of calories for each meal makes it unnecessary to keep a running calorie tally for an entire day. Instead, you only need to monitor the number of calories eaten at each meal – and there are ways to keep even this to a minimum by utilizing a concept called "Set Meals."

A set meal is a food serving that is almost identical in nutritional content and calorie count day after day. Any meal during the day that is completely under your control is a Set Meal candidate. For instance, suppose you prepare breakfast at home almost every day. Plan perhaps three set breakfasts. One might be based on cereal and fruit, another on eggs and toast, and so on. Variety is obtained by having more than one choice for a Set Meal, and by eating different kinds of cereal, or fruit, or egg preparations (scrambled, soft-boiled, etc.) – all within the same Set Meal. Once this is done, the number of calories in the Set Meal can easily calculated. Then, try to plan set meals for your mid-day meal. The more Set Meals you have in a day, the less calorie counting. For example, if you have set meals for breakfast and your mid-day meal, you only have to monitor the calories you consume at the evening meal.

Keep a Log of What You Eat

Behaviour research indicates that dieters who keep a record of what they eat generally have more successful outcomes. How should you go about this? Keep a food log. A sample Daily Food is shown in Table 6.18 with only one of the two days filled in. The slimmer's goal was 1200 kcalories.

You can keep your food log in a small notebook, a daily planner, a spreadsheet on your laptop, a pocket PC, handheld organizer, whatever works best for you. As shown, you should record the date, meal, food eaten, amount, calorie estimate, total calories for the day and any comments. To estimate the weight of a portion or serving use either a small scale or visually estimate the weight by employing guides such as 80 grams of meat or fish is about the size of a deck of cards, and 40 grams of cheese is similar in size to a pair of dice. Once you know the weight, use either Table 5.6, "Rank (kcalories per 100 grams) of Common Foods" (on page 107), or a more comprehensive calorie chart to determine the calories in a particular portion.

Log is shown in Table 6.18 with only one of the two days filled in. The slimmer's goal was 1200 kcalories. The actual total for the day was 1235 kcalories. Not bad!

You can keep your food log in a small notebook, a daily planner, a spreadsheet on your laptop, a Smart phone, handheld organizer, whatever works best for you. As shown, you should record the date, meal, food eaten,

Day	Meal	Foods	Amount	kcalories	Comments
Monday 07/10	Breakfast	Juice Cereal Skim milk Black coffee	125 mL 30 g 125 mL	55 110 40	Orange juice Wheaties
	Snack	Tea		0	
	Mid-day Meal	Cottage cheese Broccoli Whole-wheat bread	225 g 50 g 1 slice	160 25 75	Fat free
	Snack	Tea & Cracker		60	
	Evening Meal	Salmon Baked potato Green salad + olive oil Mixed vegetables Apple	125 g Medium 15 mL 50 g Medium 1 slice 250 mL	200 100 140 40 75 75 80	**Total of 1235**
	Snack	Tea		0	
Tuesday 07/11	Breakfast				
	Snack				
	Mid-day				
	Snack				
	Evening				
	Snack				

Table 6.18: Sample Daily Food Log

amount, calorie estimate, total calories for the day and any comments. To estimate the weight of a portion or serving use either a small scale or visually estimate the weight by employing guides such as 80 grams of meat or fish is about the size of a deck of cards, and 40 grams of cheese is similar in size to a pair of dice. Once you know the weight, use either Table 5.6, "Rank (kcalories per 100 grams) of Common Foods" (on page 107), or a more comprehensive calorie chart to determine the calories in a particular portion.

Graph (or Plot) Your Weight Loss: A technique to help you track your weight loss progress, is to graphically compare your actual weight loss to your expected weight loss from the appropriate Weight Loss Prediction table. If you have computer skills you can plot your weight loss on your computer using a graphical software package. Otherwise, just use ordinary graph paper. Either way proceed as follows.

First, from the Weight Loss Prediction Table appropriate for your gender, age, and activity level, choose your diet calorie level. Next, using the data in the table, plot your predicted weight loss versus time on the diet. Draw a solid line through the data points. This is your baseline against which you will compare your actual weight loss. Weigh in at the start of your diet. Then, once a week, weigh yourself first thing in the morning and plot the value. If your weight loss is less than the predicted values, either you are cheating (eating more than your diet calorie allowance), or you're not as active as the Weight Loss Prediction Table you are using requires – or both.

Weight Maintenance - Keeping It Off

Within five years, more than 90 percent of all dieters regain every pound they have lost. Why? In most instances it is because after losing weight most people eventually revert to their pre-diet eating and exercising habits, and this inevitably leads to their regaining the weight they lost – and often more. The fact is the less we weigh, the less we need to eat to sustain that lower weight. The quantity of food energy required to <u>maintain</u> a particular weight is again a function of sex, age, weight and activity level, as is clearly shown in Weight Maintenance Tables 6.19 (on page 133).

<u>Example 6.3:</u> Let's consider a 53-year-old relatively inactive female who weighed 15 stone at the start of her slimming diet. After losing 2 stone she, of course, weighed 13 stone. Determine her weight maintenance calories before and after she lost weight.

From Table 6.19 (on page 133) you find that before she started her diet, when she weighed 15 stone, her weight maintenance level was 2789 kcalories, meaning she must have been eating about 2789 kcalories of food per day. After her diet, the same table shows that in order to maintain her lower weight of 13 stone she must restrict her food intake in the future to 2550 kcalories per day. On average, to neither gain nor lose weight at 13 stone she must eat about (2789 - 2550 = 239) kcalories per day less than she did when she weighed 15 stone.

This person could help her cause by engaging in some form of exercise everyday. For example, if she walked 45 minutes every day at moderate 5.5 kph pace (covering a distance of slightly more than 4 kilometres), she could eat an additional (360 − 106) x 45 / 60 = 191 kcalories per day without gaining weight. (See Table 4.1 "Energy Expended per Hour for Different Activities" on page 36 as well as the example on page 35.)

Weight Control is a Life-Long Battle

A study, published in a 2005 issue of the Annals of Internal Medicine, that followed 4,000 people for three decades suggests that in the long term, 90 percent of men and 70 percent of women will become overweight (with a BMI ≥ 25). Interestingly, half of the men and women in the study who had made it well into adulthood without a weight problem ultimately also became overweight and a third became obese (with a BMI ≥ 30). The message is that you can never become complacent. **You must continually watch your weight because everyone is at risk of becoming overweight**.

When reach your mid to late twenties, you slowly start to lose muscle and add fat as part of the natural aging process. But muscle is metabolically active tissue. This means that your muscles use calories when they work, as well as when they repair and refuel. Fat, on the other hand, requires very few calories to exist. This is one of the reasons you need fewer calories to remain at the same weight as you get older.

In weight maintenance, it is the number of calories you eat over the long term that is important. As an illustration, the weight maintenance value of 2550 kcal per day for the 53-year-old woman in Example 6.3 amounts to about 930,750 Calories in a single year. Now realize that an annual error of only two percent of this total (that is roughly 18,600 kcal per year, or 51 Calories per day) would result in a weight gain of slightly more than 5 pounds in one year, and the importance of knowing and adhering to your personal weight maintenance calorie value becomes apparent. In brief, **to control your weight it is the number of calories eaten over the long term that matters.**

WEIGHT MAINTENANCE CALORIES FOR WOMEN

Weight (stone)	Age: 18-35 years		Age: 36-55 years		Age: 56-75 years	
	Relatively Inactive	Moderately Active	Relatively Inactive	Moderately Active	Relatively Inactive	Moderately Active
7.0	1863	2017	1761	1915	1688	1842
7.5	1938	2103	1833	1998	1758	1923
8.0	2011	2187	1903	2080	1826	2002
8.5	2083	2270	1972	2160	1893	2080
9.0	2154	2352	2040	2239	1959	2157
9.5	2223	2432	2107	2316	2024	2233
10.0	2291	2512	2173	2393	2088	2308
10.5	2359	2590	2238	2469	2151	2382
11.0	2425	2667	2302	2544	2213	2455
11.5	2491	2744	2365	2618	2274	2528
12.0	2556	2820	2427	2692	2335	2599
12.5	2620	2895	2489	2764	2395	2671
13.0	2683	2969	2550	2837	2455	2741
13.5	2746	3043	2611	2908	2514	2811
14.0	2808	3116	2671	2979	2572	2881
14.5	2869	3188	2730	3049	2630	2950
15.0	2930	3260	2789	3119	2688	3018
15.5	2990	3332	2847	3189	2745	3086
16.0	3050	3403	2905	3258	2801	3154
17.0	3169	3543	3020	3394	2913	3287
18.0	3285	3682	3133	3529	3023	3420

Table 6.19: Weight Maintenance Calories for Women

Obviously, it would be impossible for the woman in Example 6.3 to eat exactly 2550 kcalories day after day. Errors are inevitable and experience has shown that when people err they do so on the high side. They consume more calories than their maintenance value, rarely less. To allow for occasional overeating it is recommended that you plan to eat about seven percent below the values in the maintenance tables, or for the female in Example 6.3 about 2370 kcalories per day rather than the 2550 kcalories shown in the weight maintenance table – leaving her room for occasional overeating, or a missed exercise session.

Planning Weight Maintenance Eating Patterns

Once you are at your "best weight," or achieve a weight you are comfortable with, maintenance begins. Weight maintenance is in fact more difficult than being on a weight-loss diet. Why? Chiefly because maintenance requires a life-long commitment, a commitment to a new life style where you eat balanced nutritious meals that are within your maintenance calorie allowance.

Obviously, any motivational speech made at this point is not going to be much help five and ten years from now – when I trust you will still be in maintenance mode. Understand that if you really want to keep off the weight you have lost you will have to practice a good deal of self-discipline for a long time. Even the well motivated, however, need a good plan to succeed. The following approach (which is very similar to that discussed in the preceding "Planning Weight Loss Eating Patterns") is recommended:

1) Use Table 6.19 (on page 139) to determine your daily weight-maintenance calorie allowance.

2) Then decide on a weekly routine, i.e., how your calorie allowance is to be distributed among the days of the week. (As stated previously our caloric intake need not be the same for every day of the week.)

3) Next allocate the daily caloric allowance among the meals of the day according to your eating habits.

Obviously, a detailed meal plan for every possible kcalorie level cannot be included here, but given the information covered so far (particularly the food choice guidelines in Table 5.5 on page 98) it should be possible to plan eating patterns you can live with for any weight maintenance calorie allowance. (See the example that follows immediately). Granted this will take some work but in the long run it will be time well spent.

Maintenance Eating Plan Example

Example 6.4: Devise a maintenance eating plan for a 58-year-old woman who, after losing 2 stone, weighs 12st 7lb. She describes her activity level as relatively inactive. She is a semi-retired engineering consultant and works from an office in her home.

First, from table 6.19 (on page 133), we find that her maintenance calorie level is 2395 kcalories. To determine how many calories per day she should plan to consume, we deduct seven percent from 2395 to allow for occasional overeating (or under-exercising). The result is about 2205 kcal per day – the number of kcalories she should plan on eating most days. Then, we have to establish the meals she has control over (these will be her set meals), and also account for the foods she likes and dislikes. Because on most days she is home all day, she has control over every meal except evening meal. (When her husband gets home from work, they prepare the evening meal together or go out to eat.)

For breakfast the woman in Example 6.4 likes cereal (with skim or soy milk) or eggs, and for her mid-day meal she prefers a tuna sandwich, soup or cereal (if she hasn't already had cereal for breakfast). She also enjoys a morning and afternoon snack. Now we are ready to layout her meal plan for every day of the week. The resulting maintenance eating plan is broadly outlined in Table 6.21. Next, we calculate the number of calories in the foods comprising her Set Meals, i.e., her breakfasts, mid-day meals and snacks. The details behind Table 6.21 are in a spreadsheet not shown in this book.

	Monday	Tuesday	Wednesday	Thursday	Friday	Saturday	Sunday
Breakfast	Cereal (M)	Toast	Egg	Cereal (M)	Egg	Cereal (M)	Egg
Morning Snack	Fruit	Yogurt & Fruit	Yogurt & Fruit	Fruit	Yogurt & Fruit	Fruit	Yogurt & Fruit
Mid-day Meal	Soup	Cereal (S)	Cereal (S)	Tuna	Cereal (S)	Tuna	Cereal (S)
Afternoon Snack	Nuts & Seeds	Nuts & Seeds	Nuts & Seeds	Nuts & Seeds	Nuts & Seeds	Nuts & Seeds	Nuts & Seeds
Total kcal	1175	955	1075	1100	1075	1100	1075

Table 6.21: Sample Maintenance Eating Plan

For the evening meal, her calorie allowance is her maintenance kcalories minus the kcalories she has already eaten for breakfast, mid-day meal and snacks. However, from Table 6.21 we notice that her kcalorie total for breakfast, mid-day meal and snacks is not the same for every day of the week. This is not unexpected.

Because it is impractical to assign a different evening meal calorie target for every day of the week, we average the daily totals for breakfast, her mid-day meal and snacks (as shown in the worksheet), and use the average value to calculate her allowable calories for her evening meal. From Table 6.22 we see that she is allowed 1000 kcalories for her evening meal.

This evening meal calorie total should satisfy the appetite of the woman in Example 6.4 and should be easy to stay within provided she eats well-balanced meals with "reasonable" portion sizes. To understand what "reasonable" portion sizes should look like for a 1000-kcalorie meal, at first she will probably have to count calories at her evening meal. After a few weeks of counting evening-meal calories, however, she should be able to judge what is and what is not an acceptable portion size for the different foods on her plate – without actually counting calories. Using this technique, the she only has to judge or estimate her evening-meal calories to assure that she is close to her maintenance calories on a weekly basis. Once again, if you are not sure you can devise your own weight maintenance eating plan, seek the professional advice of a registered dietician.

How should she manage the inevitable, i.e., when she has to attend a business luncheon, or an all-day business meeting, or she goes on a vacation? In other words, how should she handle those days when she just can't follow her weight maintenance eating plan? First of all, she knows that her maintenance eating pattern is <u>approximately</u> 400 kcalories for breakfast, 500 kcalories for mid-day meal, 200 for snacks, 1000 kcalories for her evening meal and 250 kcalories for dessert. And if she has been following this pattern for some time, she should be able to recognize the kinds of food and the amounts (portion sizes) that make up the calories she is allowed at each meal. Then with the added understanding of how to estimate the calorie content of various foods (see page 107), she should be able to eat meals that approximate the calorie content of her weight maintenance eating plan. Lastly, if this approach does not work for her, she should realize that a day or two off her maintenance eating regimen is not the end of the world.

Use Mini Diets to Maintain Weight Loss

Many people go through life maintaining their weight without thinking about how much they eat or exercise. When they occasionally eat a bigger meal, they seem to automatically eat less at the next meal or they exercise more, or they do both. If for some reason they expend more energy, they instinctively eat more. These people are able to maintain an almost constant weight without any effort. For most of us, however, weight control is more difficult, and we must be vigilant - for us weight control is a relentless life-long challenge.

When on a when slimming diet, you should check and record your progress by weighing yourself at the same time two or three days per week. Once you are in weight maintenance mode, i.e., you have reached your desired weight level, measure your weight about once a week. Small, natural weight fluctuations can be ignored, but action is called for if you experience a "noteworthy" increase in weight.

What is a noteworthy weight gain? For a person weighing 9 stone a half-stone increase would be noteworthy; whereas for a 15-stone individual a one-stone weight gain would be noteworthy. Both would signal a call to action. Incidentally, for most people, over a lifetime, noteworthy weight shifts are all but inevitable. Nevertheless, you should consider a noteworthy weight change a warning that you may be losing control of your weight and that you need to intervene to head off a potentially significant weight gain.

If you need to lose a half stone, or a stone, to get back to your best weight, go on a short-term mini diet. Revisit the Weight Loss Prediction tables (on pages 117 to 122) and determine the calorie level needed to lose about two pounds per week. For example, a 40-year-old moderately active female weighing 9 stone, should be able to lose half a stone in approximately 27 days on a 1200 kcalorie diet, and a 40-year-old moderately active 15-stone male should be able to lose one stone in approximately 38 days on a 1800-kcalorie diet.

Once back to your best weight, revisit and analyze your weight maintenance eating and exercise routines and make any adjustments needed to keep your weight on track. Furthermore, realize that in order to maintain a proper weight level you may have to go on a number of short-term mini diets over your lifetime to correct small weight maintenance calorie eating errors.

Summarize Your Nutritional Needs

It's a good idea to summarize your nutritional needs. That way you'll have in one place the number of calories, and the nutrient and micronutrient amounts you should be eating on a daily basis. How to go about accomplishing this is again best illustrated by an example.

<u>Example 6.5</u>: Summarize the nutritional needs of a healthy 45-year old female who weighs 10 stone and describes herself as moderately active after work. She is in weight maintenance mode.

This person's nutritional needs include hers maintenance calories, the amount of protein and fat grams she should consume, and the micronutrient (vitamin and mineral) requirements specific to her age and gender. All this is shown in Table 6.22 on the next page.

For each entry, the amount, the basis for the amount, the page where the basis is found, and the food source are documented. For instance, the entry for vitamin A lists the amount (RDA) as 900 mcg; the basis as Table 5.3 on page 90; and the food sources as orange-coloured fruit and vegetables.

Please note that the cited food sources are what this particular 45-year old woman selected based on her specific needs and dietary habits. (In our opinion her choices lack plant-based protein foods such as beans and soy.)

For easy reference, make a chart similar to Table 6.22 for yourself and put on your refrigerator door, or better yet carry it with you in your briefcase, cell phone, PC, handheld organizer, or whatever works for you.

	Amount	Basis	Page	Food Source (Notes)
Weight (stone)	10	---	---	---
Total kcal	2393	Table 6.19	133	---
Protein (g)	50	0.79 gm/kg	80	---
Max Total Fat (g)	80	30%	88	Fat gm = 0.30*kcalories/9
Max Saturated Fat	27	10%	88	Fat gm = 0.10*kcalories/9
Omega-3 (g)	--	---	87	Fish 2 to 3 times per week
Fibre (g)	25	---	106	Cereal, whole-grain bread
A (mcg)	900	Table 5.3	90	Orange-coloured fruit &
D (mcg)	5	Table 5.3	90	Milk & yogurt
E (mcg)	15	Table 5.3	90	Nuts & seeds
K (mcg)*	120	Table 5.3	90	Easy to get from balanced
C (mg)	90	Table 5.3	90	180 mL orange juice
B$_1$ (mg)	1.2	Table 5.3	90	Fortified cereal
B$_2$ (mg)	1.3	Table 5.3	90	Fortified cereal
B$_3$ (mg)	16	Table 5.3	90	Fortified cereal
B$_5$ (mg)	5	Table 5.3	90	Fortified cereal
B$_6$ (mg)	1.3	Table 5.3	90	Fortified cereal
B$_7$ (mcg)	30	Table 5.3	90	Multi-vitamin & mineral
B$_9$ (mcg)	400	Table 5.3	90	Fortified cereal
B$_{12}$ (mcg)	2.4	Table 5.3	90	Fortified cereal
Calcium (mg)	1000	Table 5.4	94	Milk & dark-green
Chromium (mcg)	35	Table 5.4	94	Fortified cereal & peanut
Copper (mcg)	900	Table 5.4	94	Multi-vitamin & mineral
Fluoride (mg)	4	Table 5.4	94	Fluorinated water
Iodine (mcg)	150	Table 5.4	94	Fish 2 to 3 times per week
Iron (mg)	8	Table 5.4	94	Fortified cereal
Magnesium (mg)	420	Table 5.4	94	Dark-green-leafy
Manganese (mg)	2.3	Table 5.4	94	Multi-vitamin & mineral
Molybdenum (mcg)	45	Table 5.4	94	Multi-vitamin & mineral
Phosphorus (mg)	700	Table 5.4	94	Milk, yogurt & fish
Potassium (mg)	4700	Table 5.4	94	Bananas, oranges & leafy
Selenium (mcg)	55	Table 5.4	94	Fish 2 to 3 times per week
Zinc (mg)	11	Table 5.4	94	Fortified cereal

Table 6.22: Nutritional Needs of the Woman in Example 6.5

7. LIFE-LONG FITNESS

There are lots of reasons to get fit: a longer life expectancy, less illness, a healthful appearance, the ability to work (and play) with vigour and an energy reserve for emergencies. To repeat what was said earlier, people who undertake a physical fitness programme and attain a heightened level of fitness, report a dramatic reduction in chronic fatigue, an improved ability to relax, more energy for day-to-day tasks, firmer muscles and increased strength. In short, they feel better and look better too!

Why then is it so easy to become a dropout when fitness offers such wonderful health benefits? A fitness plan may be the missing link to getting and staying fit. Dr. Kanaar was a wonderful swimmer. He not only taught me to be a more efficient swimmer, but at the same time he convinced me that it was especially **important for an individual starting a physical fitness programme to set goals, have a plan and keep a fitness log.**

Set Goals, Have a Plan & Keep a Log

Everyone's personal goals and plan of attack will be different. Let us assume your goals are to lose one stone and improve your overall health and fitness. First, commit yourself and start immediately. (Buy a notebook, or use your cell phone, because you will need to put your goals and plans in writing.) Next, plan how you are going to attain these goals. Broadly speaking, your overall plan might be to stop smoking; to begin a weight loss diet; and to start exercising. You must, however, be more specific and develop a detailed plan that indicates the when and how you are going to stop smoking, lose weight, etcetera. You might make up your mind to stop smoking immediately, or in a month, or to enter a smoking secession programme. Note the date you plan to start and the date you expect to be smoke free. Put it in writing!

For the weight loss portion of your plan, decide if you are going to go it alone or join some sort of clinical or non-clinical slimming diet. [All the information you need for a do-it-yourself weight loss programme starts on page 111 in this book.] If you settle on a do-it-yourself programme, again note the diet calorie level, milestone dates for weight loss, etcetera. Put it in writing! Then choose an exercise routine. Again using the principles covered in this book devise a realistic plan with time, place, type of exercise and frequency. Put it writing!

By now you must appreciate why you need a notebook. Once you actually start implementing your plan, you should also keep an exercise log and a food log to record your progress. An all-in-one fitness log that includes exercise as well as food is illustrated in Table 7.1 on the next page. As you progress, periodically update your fitness plan. Enlist the support of your family and friends and do not forget to reward yourself when you reach a objective – for a job well done!

The Keys to Life-Long Fitness

As with most pursuits, the earlier in life you begin the better. But regardless of your age, the sooner you start a fitness programme the easier it will be to get in shape and the more time you will have to reap the benefits. So, for less illness, for a longer life expectancy, for a healthful appearance, start on the path to physical fitness now!

Despite all the detailed information presented in this book the path to life-long fitness is actually deceptively simple, and can be reduced to five basic keys. Assuming you have had a medical check-up, the five basic keys to life-long fitness are:

Key 1: Stop smoking and limit the consumption of alcoholic beverages. For some this will be difficult but both are absolutely necessary for life-long fitness.

Key 2: Keep your weight under control. Know your maintenance calorie value, i.e., how many calories you can eat to neither gain nor lose weight. Periodically you might experience a noteworthy weight gain. If this happens go on a mini-diet.

Key 3: Practice good nutrition by eating a variety of foods from each food group – all within your caloric allowance.

Key 4: Engage in some form of moderate strength training at least two non-consecutive days per week.

Key 5: Engage in some form of moderate aerobic exercise every single day of the year. That is right every day! (If need be, cut back your aerobic workout on the days you do your strength exercises.)

To repeat, make every effort to engage in some form of moderate aerobic exercise every single day of the year! And try to exercise at the same time every day. This will probably mean rearranging priorities and putting exercise close to the top of your list. Soon exercise will become a part of your daily routine and you will not feel right unless you have had your daily run, or daily walk, etcetera.

Meal	Foods	Amount	kcalories	Comments
Breakfast	Juice Cereal Skim milk Black coffee	125 mL 30 g 125 mL	55 110 40	Orange Juice Wheat cereal
Snack	Tea		0	
Mid-day Meal	Cottage cheese Broccoli Whole wheat bread	225 g 50 g 1 slice	160 25 75	Fat free
Snack	Cracker or biscuit Tea		60	
Evening Meal	Salmon Baked potato Green salad + olive oil Mixed veggies Apple Whole wheat bread Skim milk	125 g Medium 15 mL 50 g Medium 1 slice 250 mL	200 100 140 40 75 75 80	Total of 1235 kcal
Snack	Tea		0	

Strength Exercise	Dumbbell Weight	Reps	Sets	Aerobic Exercise	Distance	Time	Heart Rate
Bench Press	5 kg	12	2	Walking	6.75 km	72mi	124
Rows	7 kg	12	2				
Tricep Ext	5 kg	12	2				
Press	5 kg	12	2				
Curls	7 kg	12	2				
Squats	7 kg	10	1				
Abs	N/A	25	2				

Table 7.1: Sample All-In-One Fitness Log for Tuesday July 11th

Yes, there will be some days when it will be impossible to fit exercise into your schedule – but those days should be the exception and should be few and far between. Any other occasional additional exercise such as a round of golf, a game of handball, cross-country skiing, attending a yoga class, is fine, beneficial, but should be considered secondary to your daily aerobic workout.

Make It Happen

At this point, you have everything you need to succeed. You have an understanding of the fundamentals of exercise, nutrition and weight control. You have set realistic fitness goals, and you have a good fitness plan. If you combine all these with intense desire you'll be unstoppable. Your fitness regimen will work wonders and will have you looking and feeling better both physically and mentally. And when you look and feel your best, your spirit will soar.

So as you start on the road to fitness, be aware that you are well prepared for success and always keep in mind how good you'll feel when you reach your goals.

So what are you waiting for? Make it happen!

Good luck!

Disclaimer: This book offers general fitness information. It is not a medical manual and the author does not claim to be medically qualified. The material in this book is not intended to be a substitute for medical counselling. Everyone should have a medical check-up before beginning a physical fitness program (whether the program involves weight loss, nutritional changes, or exercise). Moreover, the physician conducting the medical exam should be made aware of and should approve the specific physical fitness routine planned. Additionally, while the author and publisher have made every effort to ensure the accuracy of the information in this book, they make no representations or warranties regarding its accuracy or completeness. Further, the reader is cautioned that all fitness programmes include some risk of injury or illness. Neither the author nor publisher assume liability for any medical problems that might result from applying the methods in this book, or for any loss of profit, or any other commercial damages, including but not limited to special, incidental, consequential or other damages, and any such liability is hereby expressly disclaimed.

Vincent W. Antonetti, Ph.D., is an emeritus professor at Manhattan College.

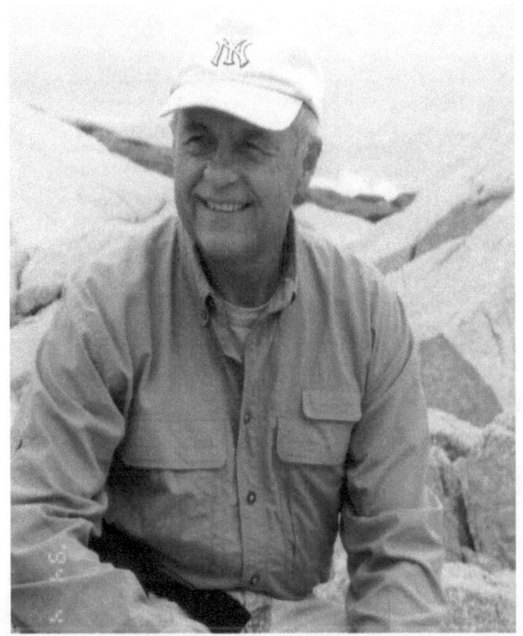

He has been a lecturer at IBM Management and Professional Development classes and often speaks to groups on fitness and weight control. He is an expert in the mathematics and thermodynamics of weight control. Among his many publications is the highly regarded, "The Equations Governing Weight Change in Human Beings," published by The *American Journal of Clinical Nutrition.* And Dr. Antonetti's critically acclaimed book *The Computer Diet* was given *Consumer Guide* magazine's highest rating. He is a life-long exercise and nutrition enthusiast, and although a senior citizen he still maintains a vigorous physical fitness program.

Photographed while hiking in Nova Scotia, Canada